Yoga with a

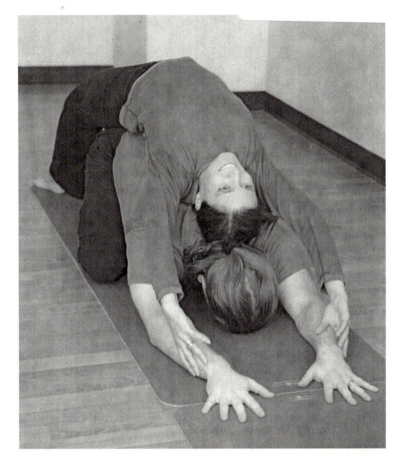

Develop trust, communication, strength, and compassion when you practice yoga with a partner

By Kimberlee Jensen Stedl and Todd Stedl, Ph.D.

Published by 8th Element Yoga, a division of
8th Element Recreation LLC
1916 Pike Place
Suite 12-440
Seattle, WA 98101

Published in Seattle, Washington, USA.

Printed in the United States of America.

First edition: December 2007

ISBN 978-0-6151-8318-3

Visit us on the Web at www.8thElementYoga.com

To my husband, for helping me grow into a better person each day.

To my wife, whose love gives me the courage to explore bold ideas.

Acknowledgements

We would like to thank Down Dog Missoula for all their support of Kimberlee's partner yoga class and for use of the studio for our photo sessions. We would also like to thank Planet Earth Yoga, for being a great yoga studio host for our workshops in Seattle. Thank you to all of the students who attended our workshops. We have enjoyed learning from you as much as we enjoyed teaching you.

Kimberlee would like to thank all of her yoga teachers and teacher-trainers who have taught her. She would also like to thank all of her students who attended Punk Rock Yoga classes over the years and were willing and open to try all the crazy partner yoga poses she threw at them.

Todd would like to thank Kimberlee and the other yoga teachers he's had, for encouraging him and being patient with him. Yoga has benefited him both mentally and physically and he would not have pursued it without their help.

We would like to thank Christopher Williams for taking the pose and tango dance shots in this book. Christopher is a true professional with a great eye. We also thank Alex Crick for helping us with our workshop handouts that helped build the foundation for this book and for contributing the photo of us used on the cover. We greatly appreciate yoga instructor Sylvia Demaras for being our technical consultant during the pose photo shoot. Her help and alignment guidance was invaluable. We would like to thank fellow yoga instructor Becca Powell for her tremendous help in proofreading this book and for her suggestions to improve its content. We would also like to thank Elizabeth Worcester and Jeff Simpson for the photo of us at our wedding that we used in the About the Authors section.

Finally, we would like to thank our families and friends for their wonderful support of our marriage. We thank everyone who flew thousands of miles for our wedding, along with everyone else who throughout the years have supported our union.

Table of Contents

Disclaimer

This book is for self-knowledge and is not a substitute for consulting with a physician or physical therapist. Please consult your physician before beginning a new physical conditioning program, especially if you have a pre-existing condition for which you are being treated or you have been inactive for a long period of time. All the poses in this book assume the reader is physically capable of these poses; however they do carry risks and only you and your health care providers can say what poses work and do not work for your body at this point in time.

Women who are pregnant must consult with their physician before practicing yoga poses and are advised to take a pre-natal yoga class instead of doing a general yoga practice. People recovering from injuries should consult with their doctor or their physical therapist as certain poses may aggravate an injury and delay healing. We strongly advise taking this book with you to your physicians and asking them to select the appropriate poses for you, especially if you have a known condition for which you see a physician or take medication regularly.

The best portion of a good man's life: his little, nameless, unremembered acts of kindness and love.

—William Wordsworth

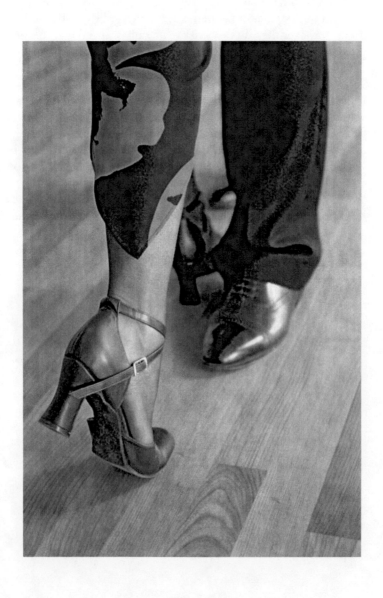

Introduction

Practicing yoga with a friend creates a new dynamic. You use yoga not only to connect with your own body and mind, but also to connect with someone else. We have found that practicing together helps us maintain a healthy marriage. In fact, when outside stresses get the best of us, we find that practicing yoga together helps us draw strength from our union and better enables us to show gratitude for having each other in our lives.

Sharing your practice with a partner is an act of *aparigraha* (non-greediness). If you have been practicing solo for years, it may take some time to adapt, but you will soon find its rewards. We believe this practice has all the normal benefits of yoga: strength, flexibility, peacefulness, and mindfulness, but adds another dimension of developing compassion for and empathy with your friend.

Numerous yoga styles abound. In this book, we have approached the poses from the *Hatha* yoga philosophy. *Hatha* fuses the words for sun and moon in Sanskrit and it essentially means balancing aggressive sun energy with receptive moon energy. In your physical pose practice, you do this by doing both vigorous poses, such as Two Sided Plank, and relaxing poses, such as Open Cobbler's. *Hatha* yoga is also an umbrella term for numerous other styles. In addition, we applied some principles of *Vinyasa* yoga, which denotes flowing from pose to pose with the breath. *Vinyasa* yoga is a subset of *Hatha* yoga.

In fact, we view practicing with a partner as a great way to balance aggressive and receptive energy, which is the essence of *Hatha* yoga. When two people practice together, both bring a combination of masculine and feminine qualities to each pose. One partner might bring more strength while the other brings more flexibility, so when they practice together they can harmonize those two characteristics—the stronger partner helps the other gain strength while the more flexible partner helps the other stretch more.

For couples, practicing the poses together helps develop great intimacy, but without the pressure and emotional charge of sex. However, *Yoga with a Friend* is not only just for couples, but also for friends and family to practice together. It's a wonderful way to spend quality time together, strengthening and opening both physically and emotionally.

In partner poses, you can experience the wonder of non-verbal communication and shared commonalities. This is the essence of the word *namaste*, which many teachers say at the end of yoga classes. *Namaste* has been translated in so many ways, but essentially it means, "I honor the place in your soul that has the same inherent goodness and light as I find in my own soul." So every time you hold a pose with a friend, you open a window into what you have in common—your basic humanity. In practicing these partner poses, you truly put meaning into the word *namaste*.

If you practice yoga regularly on your own, you will notice several immediate differences in practicing with a partner. Instead of practicing your favorite poses, you will probably practice some poses you do less frequently as you and your friend negotiate your pose sequence. Initially, you will speak more than in a solo practice, but through time you will learn to adjust to each pose intuitively. The more you practice with your partner the more you will create this balance non-verbally. Over time, you and your practice mate will develop great awareness of subtle adjustments to make, but without speaking. Enjoy the process and remember to have a good laugh if you stumble out of a pose.

Our goal with *Yoga with a Friend* is to help you use yoga as a tool for growth in all your relationships. With the physical poses, we hope to share some great ideas for turning traditionally solitary yoga poses into fun and challenging partner poses. We did not want to impress you with extraordinary acrobatics, but rather demonstrate some poses that people with an average level of strength and flexibility can do together.

We do not recommend that you replace your existing yoga practice with partner yoga but rather that you diversify your practice to incorporate partner poses. We provide suggestions for how to do this later in this book.

Of course, the poses are just a part of overall yoga philosophy. In this book, we briefly introduce the other seven limbs of the eight-limbed royal yoga philosophy. We explore some of the behavioral guidelines and how you can apply them to build healthy relationships.

We also included some guided visualizations that can help you not only strengthen your relationships with the people in your life, but also help you strengthen your own sense of self and build your self-esteem. Visualizations are a powerful meditative tool, and we invite you to begin exploring with our suggestions. Enjoy the journey!

What is yoga?

Yoga is one of six ancient Indian philosophies dating back more than 5,000 years. Even though many people consider yoga merely stretching and breathing exercises, it goes far beyond that. Yoga is primarily psychological and spiritual development. Yoga is not a religion and does not prescribe a belief system to you, but through practicing meditation and other aspects of yoga, you can develop a greater connection with your own spirituality. The term *yoga* in Sanskrit means to yoke, or to unify. Through yoga, you unite the body and the mind, which in the West we have often separated. You also unite your lifestyle with your belief system, whatever it may be. When practicing with a friend, you also unite your bodies and minds, as you share the experience every step of the way.

There are several braches of yoga. Most often in the West you will encounter royal *(raja)* yoga, also known as active yoga. This form of yoga is organized into eight components, called limbs. The first seven limbs are considered steps on the way to the final limb, liberation *(samadhi)*.

When people hear the word yoga, though, they generally think of only the third limb of royal yoga, which deals with physical poses *(asanas)*. Scores of books devoted to the poses fill bookshops, but ironically in the original royal yoga text, the only thing ever written about the poses is this: "*Asana* is a steady comfortable posture." *Hatha* yoga, a style of practicing poses that seeks to balance aggressive sun *(ha)* energy with receptive moon *(tha)* energy, follows the royal yoga path. In *Yoga with a Friend*, we use the principles of *Hatha* yoga.

Classically, in some traditions such as Iyengar yoga, practicing with a friend meant that you would assist your friend as he or she did a pose. For example, you would gently press your friend's hips back as he or she held a Downward Facing Dog pose. As many Western teachers began playing with the poses, they found more ways to incorporate another person into the poses, making it true partner yoga rather than merely assisted yoga. Some teachers have even started to include groups of people in one pose, such as in Acro Yoga. We find this fusion exciting! The more we create new variations that our bodies can do safely, the more we are empowered to understand the dynamics of our physical structure, including strengths and limitations.

After you have finished this book, we encourage you to craft your own pose variations. The more you practice these poses and focus on how they feel, the more able you are to realize how to move into optimal alignment for the bones and joints and how to modify poses to make them safe for you and your partner. Honesty—which is one of the yoga lifestyle guidelines we discuss later in this book—is an integral part of gaining the self-knowledge and self-confidence in creating your own partner yoga poses. The more you can be honest with yourself and with your partner about how each pose feels, the more safety you will bring to the pose practice.

An important concept in yoga is that the self is ultimately the best teacher. Traditionally in yoga study, you would read what others have written, listen to what others have said, and then spend time contemplating these ideas and forming your own conclusions. After reading this book, practicing the poses, and reflecting over the concepts, perhaps you can learn more about yourself and about your partner. We encourage you to spend time in introspection and in discussion with your partner and hope the symbolisms we describe for each pose and the philosophy concepts we introduce in *Yoga with a Friend* provide a stimulus for your discussions.

Are we practicing tantra?

Tantra is a highly complex philosophical system of Indian spirituality with numerous practices and which has been frequently misunderstood in the West. While many Indian philosophies divide the world into two camps: everything we see physically—which is often considered an illusion—and universal truth—which is often considered akin to an eternal soul—tantra takes a different approach by viewing everything we see physically as the truth.

Tantric practices involve the fusion of masculine and feminine qualities, which are viewed as a continuum. Through many rituals, the practice seeks to unite these two powers, via what tantrics consider energy channels of body. For example, the Kundalini style of yoga, which derives from tantric practices, focuses on opening energy channels in the body to tap into the root of feminine energy.

Many Westerners focus on an aspect of tantra that involves sexuality, but that is only a small component of tantric practices. The sexual rituals in tantra have nothing to do with better orgasms, but rather with attaining a sense of liberation by merging the feminine powers with the masculine powers that dwell in each of us.

Even though we strive to balance masculine and feminine qualities in the poses, *Yoga with a Friend* is not written to be a tantric practice. While the Full Circle Breathing exercise (see page 22) is based on a tantric ritual, you do not need to espouse the philosophy of tantra to benefit from the exercise. You can simply view Full Circle Breathing as a way to connect to your partner and as a way to practice a relaxing, meditative breath. The intention you bring to any endeavor truly defines it; you make the practice what you need it to be—tantric or not.

Friendship is the only thing in the world concerning the usefulness of which all mankind are agreed.

—Cicero

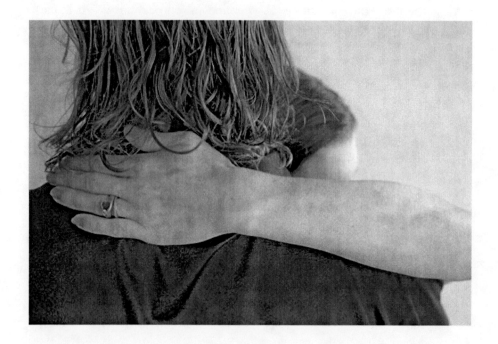

Before you practice

Despite all the advertising to the contrary, you only need a very simple setup to practice yoga. One thing we love about yoga is its portability—you can practice yoga on your living room carpet, on the beach, in a park—wherever you can find a relatively flat, smooth surface with enough softness to accommodate kneeling, but not so much that it will bend your wrists. Some people purchase a sticky mat to help keep their hands and feet in place. However, plenty of people practice without a mat.

If you do use mats for your partner yoga practice, you will sometimes have them lined up side-by-side, and other times end-to-end. The photos in *Yoga with a Friend* demonstrate suggested mat alignment. We have sequenced the poses to minimize the number of times you need to rearrange the mats, while observing a progression that warms up your muscles before proceeding to the deeper poses.

We recommend having a chair or a wall nearby for when you need additional support. Some people purchase blocks for when their hands do not reach the floor—this is an option as well. Many people use straps to help extend their reach in various poses, but you can do the same with an old necktie, a small towel, or an old stretchy sock.

You can wear simple athletic clothing to practice yoga. In India, many people practice in their regular office clothing, however we advocate wearing something without belts, buckles or zippers because those can dig into the skin. Clothing need not be skin tight, but if it is too loose it can distract you. Traditionally you would do the poses barefoot, so that you strengthen your feet and ankles while developing mechanical awareness of your stance. However, if you have foot problems and need to wear shoes, you can wear them for all of the standing poses. Most of the floor poses can be done in socks, but avoid wearing socks for the standing poses—it is too easy to slip in them.

Many yoga teachers recommend practicing yoga for one hour a day. For practicing with a friend, we recommend setting aside one hour per week, or ninety minutes per week if you want to do all the poses in this book. This will allow you to work on your own practice during the week and to view this shared practice as a treat. Consistency is more important than both intensity and duration, so evaluate your current schedule and carve out the time you can mutually allot to practice. Often, we will do our solo practice simultaneously and spend the last moments in a few partner poses. For our full partner practice, we find Sunday evenings to be our favorite time, as for us, Sunday evenings are generally free from other obligations. You can even do a couple of the more relaxing poses, and the Full Circle Breath, right before bedtime as a great way to ease into sleep.

This book is geared towards helping you create your own practice. If you are new to yoga, we highly recommend joining a weekly yoga class to learn the poses solo in addition to practicing with a partner, so that you can develop your own body awareness.

Yogic view of breath

Breathing is unique in that it's the only bodily function that is both involuntary and voluntary. Our bodies keep breathing without any conscious effort, but yet we can also consciously control our respiration. We can't do that with the beating of our heart, so our respiratory system is really unlike any other system.

Relaxed, full, steady breathing is essential to yoga. Yogis have invented several breathing exercises to master the breath. Throughout your pose practice, you can use Victorious Breath *(Ujayi Pranayama)*— long steady inhalations and exhalations with a gentle emphasis at the back of the throat. Try exhaling with a "ha" sound, and then try making the same sound with your mouth closed to produce a whispery sound, almost like a subtle snore. As you practice this breath, allow your chest and belly to expand without force as you inhale and feel your belly and chest contract as you exhale. In this book we introduce Full Circle Breath, a partner breathing exercise, which uses the same mechanics as Victorious Breath, but also requires coordination with your partner.

Breathing is the foundation of your yoga practice. Begin your session with a few minutes of Full Circle Breath to help the mind transition from focusing on what you did in the past and what you might do in the future to focusing on what you are doing in the present. When you practice Full Circle Breath, really listen to your partner's breath: it's a wonderful exercise in active listening.

Full Circle Breath with a partner, or Victorious Breath solo, can be done independent of your yoga pose session. Deep breathing exercises help prepare the body for sleep, provide you with serenity in a crisis, and provide some energy. These are great practices for anytime and anywhere.

Basic yoga guidelines

Yoga practices strive towards balance, both on a philosophical plane and a physical plane. A balanced yoga pose practice works all sides of the body as equally as possible. In structuring a yoga class, teachers focus on balancing the directional movement of the spine:

Bending forward

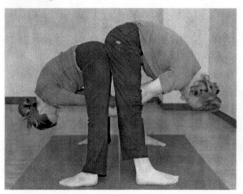

Twisting side-to-side

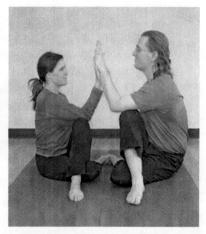

Bending backward

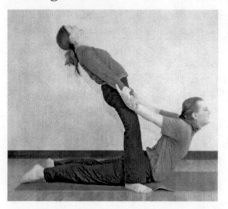

Bending side-to-side

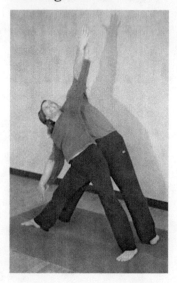

For everything you do on the right side, you also do on the left during your practice. We show many single-sided poses in this book, so make sure you do both sides. You should do a relatively equal number of forward and backward bends, and incorporate both strengthening and stretching poses for both the upper and lower body.

In terms of sequencing, you want to warm up the spine gently at first, with something like Cat/Cow with a Starfish and warm up the large muscle groups with poses such Double Down Dog. Also, you should progress naturally from the more subtle bends such as Open Hearted Warrior to deeper bends, such as Double Cobra.

In yoga, we emphasize the effort, not the final result of the practice. If you can't touch your toes today, then maybe you will tomorrow, or the next day, or the next year. The time you take to practice will benefit you, even if you never touch your toes. Our intention with the pose demonstrations is not to impress you with acrobatics, but rather to demonstrate poses that people with average strength and flexibility can do. Average does not mean everyone, so there will be some poses that come rather easily to you, and some poses that will confound you. Be patient with the process.

For some of the poses, we have provided modifications and options. As you experiment with each pose, you should find the place where you feel work, but not pain. If a pose feels painful, particularly in the joints, you should either modify the pose or skip it completely.

Many people modify poses by using a chair or a wall for support. For example, you can place one hand the wall while practicing balance poses for extra stability. Or you can place hands on the seat of the chair, instead of the floor, for many arm-strengthening poses to avoid pain in the wrists. You might also want to keep a necktie, small towel, or old sock handy to extend your arms in various stretching poses as well. It's also perfectly acceptable for just one person in your partner team to be using a wall or chair.

There is no shame in modifying poses. In fact, as both of us have dealt with various injuries over the years, we have had to modify our practice numerous times. Every body is different and the important thing is that you practice safely and stay in tune with your body throughout the practice. Yoga teaches us to heed our bodies, so we strongly recommend making all the adjustments necessary to work hard, but to work well.

Many times people tend to practice the poses that come very easy to them. Because yoga poses are a great tool for psychological growth—teaching us to overcome our fears and aversions—you should try to practice the most challenging poses too, instead of just doing the things that come easy to you. When we practice easy poses, our minds can wander to various places, but when we practice difficult poses, our minds stay with us in the practice. One great thing about working with a friend is that because everyone has different anatomical proportions, a pose that comes easily to you may not come easily to your practice mate, so you will naturally do a wider variety of poses.

Our caveat, of course, is that difficult does not mean painful. If you are healing a medical condition and have been instructed by your doctor not to do certain poses, then find other poses to do. We encourage you to try the poses that you find hard, not impossible, painful, or dangerous for your unique physical condition.

Partners of different shapes and sizes

When your practice mate is significantly taller or shorter than you, such as when you practice with a child, you will have to modify some poses to account for height differentials. For example, in Double Tree, the shorter person's arms can wrap around the other person's thighs instead of the hips. In Upright Back Chair, you can have the shorter person actually sit in a chair. You can also have the taller person practice on their knees, or at least step his or her feet further apart, making it more of a wide squat pose.

For poses that require you to support your partner's weight, you may have to modify if there are significant weight differences. For example, in Cat/Cow with a Starfish, you may have to just practice Cat/Cow as a solo pose or possibly substitute it with Child's Play.

You can use these poses to help motivate a friend or a loved-one to get in shape, but please remember to keep the conversation positive. If your practice mate has been sedentary for a while, avoid talking about their flexibility or strength issues. When you offer modifications, just say, "Let's try it this way instead," rather than drawing attention to their challenges. Focus on their progress and applaud their success.

If your practice mate is dealing with weight management issues, find poses that the two of you can do together, such as many of the standing poses. Avoid poses that only one of you can do because you can't hold your partner's weight—such as Cat/Cow with a Starfish—and substitute a side-by-side Cat/Cow instead. Focus on the poses your partner can do, rather than point out what he or she cannot do.

Positive reinforcement works much better than negative reinforcement. As you practice yoga with someone you care about, remember that practicing with a friend is above all an exercise in compassion.

What is a friend? A single soul dwelling in two bodies.

—Aristotle

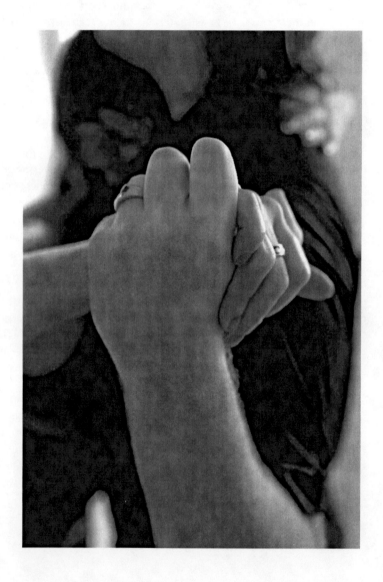

Alignment and anatomy basics

Even though practicing with a partner means making some subtle compromises in the way you practice the poses solo, here are some general alignment guidelines to follow:

- When your feet are bearing weight, such as in standing poses like Two Warriors, your kneecap should always point to your second toe and your knee should never move forward beyond your ankle.

- When your feet are weight bearing, your toes should be spread wide, and the arches of your feet should remain lifted.

- When your feet are not weight bearing, your toes should be spread wide and in many poses you will flex the foot by pressing out through the heel.

- When your hands are weight bearing, such as in poses like Double Down Dog, your fingers should be spread wide and your middle finger should face forward, so that your wrists stay straight.

- When your hands are not weight bearing, consider them as part of the pose. If the hands float freely in the air, keep extending through the fingers.

- Your shoulders should remain down away from the ears, except when you reach your arms overhead, such as in Gibbous Moon, when your shoulders will have a slight, natural lift.

- Your head should act as a natural extension to your spine. In some poses it will extend backward, such as in Double Cobra, but in that case your head is following what the rest of the spine is doing. Unless you are folding forward or bending backward, your ears should be lined up over your shoulders, which for many people means sliding the jaw back slightly.

- When you are twisting or bending to the side, your spine should still maintain neutral alignment. Avoid rounding or arching the back while twisting or bending to the side. For example, in Twister Triangle, keep your spine reasonably straight as you twist.

- When bending forward, such as in Extended Table, bend at the hip crease, instead of at the waist. This will feel like you are pushing your tailbone backward instead of pushing the middle of your back upward.

- Your abdominal muscles should engage throughout the poses to support your spinal column. This is especially true in all of the forward folding poses, such as Super Straddle, where we often just let the upper body rest. By engaging the abdominal muscles in these poses, you provide support for the joints of the lower back. This will feel like you are drawing your belly button towards your spine.

- You want your muscles to hold the body steady in the poses, rather than relying on the joints to bear the burden. The joints should stay firm, but not locked into place. You can keep a tiny bend in the joints, particularly the knees and elbows, to avoid extending them beyond a healthy range. For example, in Just Right Triangle, you should be able to feel your quadriceps muscles in the fronts of the thighs contracting and working. If not, try to lift your kneecap towards your hip to engage these muscles.

- One great test to see if you are working beyond your limits in each pose is to observe your breath. If your breath becomes short and choppy, try backing off from the pose slightly, or stop to take a break. Your breath should be smooth and steady throughout each pose.

- Our final rule on alignment is to trust your instincts and your own body. The poses should feel like your muscles are working and stretching, but if something feels super funky in a pose, it probably is. Come out of the pose, establish better alignment, and try again. If it still doesn't feel right, modify the pose or skip it altogether.

In each pose, we point out what various muscles are doing, so it's important to have a basic understanding of how our muscles work. The muscles exist to move the bones, and the joints act as the fulcrum for that movement. The tendons connect muscles to the bones, and the ligaments connect bones to other bones. Tendons and ligaments are part of your joints.

Muscles can move the joint in several ways. The first two are flexion (to decrease the angle between the bones) and extension (to increase the angle between the bones). For example, the hamstring muscles flex the knee, or bend it, and the quadriceps muscles extend the knee, or straighten it. Similarly, the biceps muscles flex the elbow joint and the triceps muscles extend the elbow joint.

Muscles can also act as rotators for the joints that move in multiple directions: numerous muscles in the shoulder and hip aid in rotation. A group of muscles in the shoulder—the supraspinatus, infraspinatus, teres minor, and subscapularis—form the rotator cuff.

Two other movement actions are adduction, which is movement toward the midline of your body, and abduction, which is movement away from the midline of your body. Primarily, the muscles of the shoulder and hip joint perform abduction and adduction.

The final action for the muscles, which is most important in yoga, is stabilization. When muscles stabilize the joint, they prevent the joint from hyperextension, which could result in both muscle tear and overstretched ligaments. Once the ligaments stretch, they weaken and they never regain their shape, which makes the joint unstable and susceptible to injury. Muscles can be both a mover and a stabilizer for a joint. For example, the rectus abdominus muscle—the large abdominal muscle in the center of your belly—both flexes the spine and stabilizes the spine.

Another concept of the muscles that is particularly important for yoga is the concept of agonist and antagonist. The agonist causes the joint to move while the antagonist opposes the move. For example, when you straighten your elbow, the triceps muscle works as the agonist or the prime mover, and the biceps muscle works as the antagonist. If your biceps are tight, then the triceps can only straighten the elbow so far. This system helps prevent the ligaments and tendons from tearing.

What actually happens during movement is that when you contract an agonist, your brain fires a message to the antagonist to relax. This is called reciprocal inhibition. So if you want to stretch your hamstring muscle, contracting the quadriceps will tell the hamstrings to relax and stretch. They will only relax as far as your flexibility allows on that day, but the more you practice yoga, the more flexible your muscles can become and the greater your range of motion you will have. Good range of motion helps prevent injury.

One great thing about yoga is that many poses require both the agonist and antagonist to contract simultaneously to stabilize the joint. In many poses, such as Double Down Dog, you contract both the erector spinae—which run along the center of the back—and the rectus abdominus to stabilize the spine in a neutral position.

Because we mention numerous muscle groups in our pose descriptions, we have included a basic muscle anatomy diagram, with the muscles we mention highlighted. There are approximately 639 muscles in the body, but we only demonstrate the muscles we most frequently mention in this book.

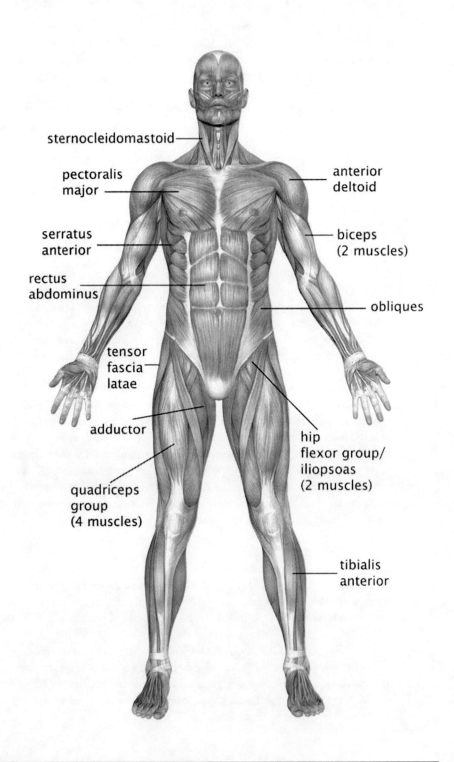

sternocleidomastoid

pectoralis
major

serratus
anterior

rectus
abdominus

tensor
fascia
latae

adductor

quadriceps
group
(4 muscles)

anterior
deltoid

biceps
(2 muscles)

obliques

hip
flexor group/
iliopsoas
(2 muscles)

tibialis
anterior

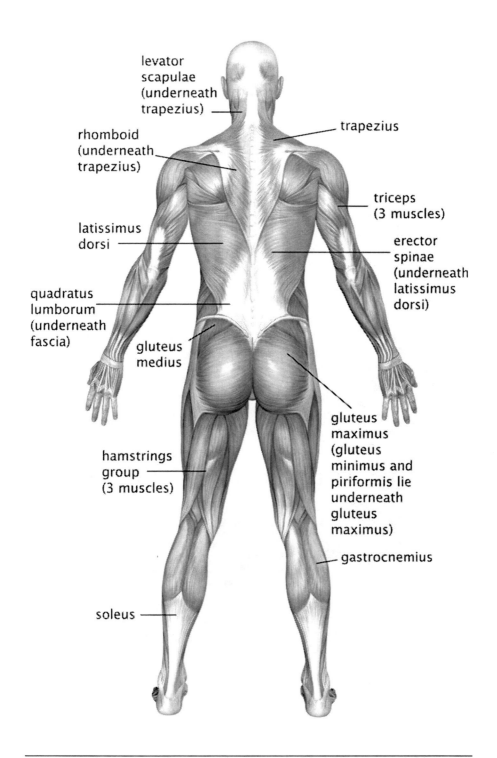

levator
scapulae
(underneath
trapezius)

rhomboid
(underneath
trapezius)

latissimus
dorsi

quadratus
lumborum
(underneath
fascia)

gluteus
medius

hamstrings
group
(3 muscles)

soleus

trapezius

triceps
(3 muscles)

erector
spinae
(underneath
latissimus
dorsi)

gluteus
maximus
(gluteus
minimus and
piriformis lie
underneath
gluteus
maximus)

gastrocnemius

Don't walk in front of me, I may not follow. Don't walk behind me, I may not lead. Just walk beside me and be my friend.

—Albert Camus

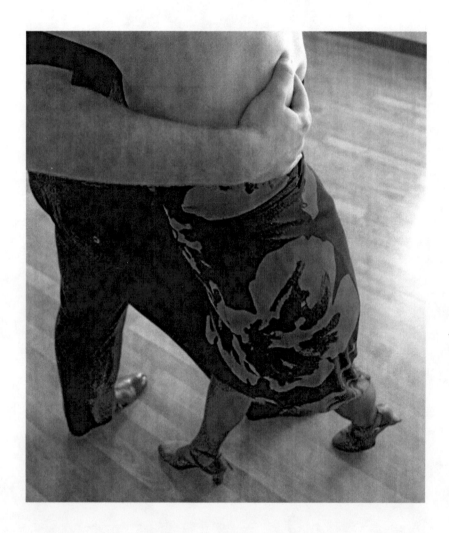

Practice sequence

We have sequenced the poses in this book for a start-to-finish practice that will take roughly ninety minutes. It will probably take longer the first several times, as you will be referring to the book throughout the sequence. Also, you can play with the sequence and customize it to suit your needs. Some days you might want to just do some seated poses for a quiet evening practice; other days you might want to just do some active standing poses for a wake-up practice.

The time duration of each pose can vary, but we recommend holding the strength-building active poses for roughly four complete cycles of Full Circle Breath, and the more relaxing stretching poses for roughly eight complete cycles of Full Circle Breath. However, some poses have a flow sequence, such as Cat/Cow with a Starfish. When you flow between poses you move with every inhalation and exhalation.

To help you connect the text with the photos, we are calling Kimberlee "Partner A" and Todd "Partner B."

Full Circle Breath

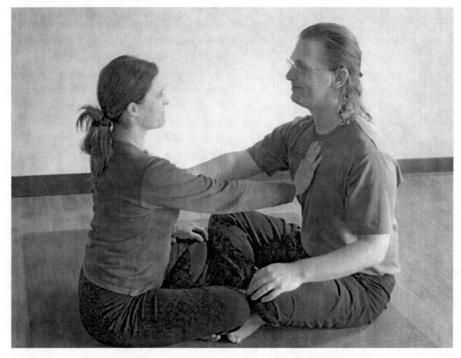

1. Begin with both partners sitting in a comfortable seated position, such as cross-legged on the floor.

2. Partners sit knee-to-knee.

3. Both partners reach one hand to touch their partner's heart.

4. As partner A inhales, partner B exhales, and vice versa, using a four-count breath of "inhale 1-2-3-4, exhale 4-3-2-1".

5. Breath moves through the nose, with a soft whispery sound at the back of the throat, as in Victorious Breath (see page 9).

6. Partners can look into each other's eyes, or keep the eyes closed.

7. Breathe like this for several minutes to begin the practice session.

By alternating breath in this way, Full Circle Breath demonstrates how partners can feed off of each other's energy. It's a wonderful experience to share the simple yet vital act of breathing. Tuning in to your friend's breath creates great harmony and empathy.

By maintaining a slow, steady rhythm in the breath, you reduce hormones that surge when you get stressed. Rhythmic breathing such as this also induces an awake, yet peaceful brain wave pattern. When both partners adhere to the four-count breath, both will be able to take full, deep, steady breaths. Counting upwards to and backwards from four also helps your mind concentrate on the practice, and allows you to temporarily set aside your concerns for the day.

This Full Circle Breath practice should be done before the poses to help bring focus into the practice and to help remind you to breath deeply and calmly throughout the practice. You can also practice this breath exercise independent of the poses, such as using it as a way to relax just before bedtime.

Symbolism: The symbolism of Full Circle Breath is the circle of life, and how what goes around does come around. This breath symbolizes a full circle, and you can visualize the breath circulating between you and your partner. This breath is also very symbolic of the give-and-take nature of healthy relationships.

This pose is derived from a tantric breathing exercise.

Full Circle OM

You can also practice OM chants with Full Circle Breath. Chanting has many positive benefits, not the least of which is that rhythmic chants reduce stress. OM is not strictly a word, but rather a sound which has many interpretations in the yoga community. We like to consider it symbolic of that which is eternal and universal.

To chant OM, you open your mouth wide for the sound of "ah", then close slightly, rounding your lips for the sound of "oh", and finally close the lips for the sound of "mmm"; when you complete the chant, listen for the echo that follows.

To practice Full Circle OM, have Partner A begin her chant of OM while Partner B inhales, then as Partner B begins his chant of OM, Partner A inhales. This practice follows a call-and-response pattern not unlike many singing traditions. After a few rounds, you create an extraordinary rhythm that sounds like a perpetual OM. It's a wonderful chant to try either at the beginning or at the end of your yoga practice.

Cat/Cow with a Starfish

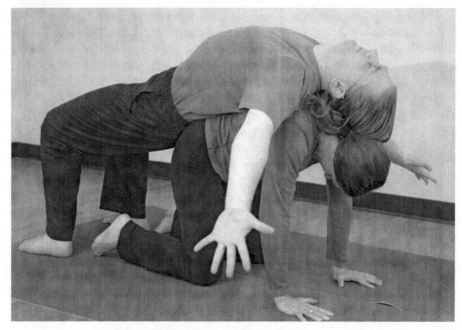

1. Partner A comes down on hands and knees, keeping her hands directly under her shoulders and her knees directly under her hips.

2. Partner A can either keep her palms flat on the floor, with fingers stretched wide and middle finger pointing forward, or make a fist with the knuckles on the floor and the palms facing inward.

3. To start, Partner A maintains a neutral spine by engaging evenly among the muscles in the front and back of the torso.

4. Partner B stands facing away from Partner A.

5. Partner B squats down, taking his hips to Partner A's hips.

6. Slowly, Partner B lies back, keeping his knees bent and his feet flat on the floor.

   - If getting into the pose proves challenging for Partner B, he can use a chair next to him for additional support as he comes in to and out of the pose.

- Another option is for Partner A to start closer to the floor, like in Child's Play (see page 82), and allow Partner B to climb on her back that way, then lifting Partner B up as she comes on to all fours.

7. Partner B opens his arms straight out to the side, letting his hands reach towards the floor.

8. Partner B lets his head rest as close to Partner A's head as possible.

9. Partner A moves into Cat by contracting the abdominal muscles strongly and rounding her back, drawing her chin and hips in towards her ribs as she exhales.

10. Partner A moves into Cow by inhaling as she arches her back, dropping the navel towards the floor and looking up as far as is comfortable.

11. Partner B enjoys a wonderful chest opener.

12. After four breath cycles of flowing through this pose, partners trade positions.

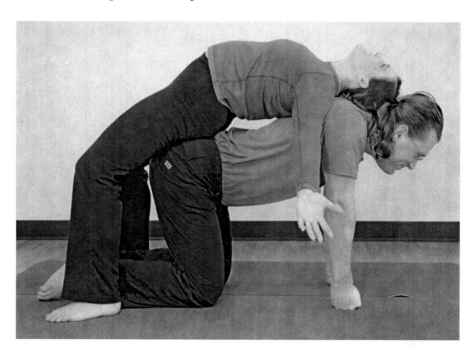

Cat/Cow with a Starfish is a wonderful backbend for the partner on top. It helps open the pectoral muscles in the chest, the rectus abdominus in the belly, and the hip flexor muscles in the front of the hips. For the partner on the bottom, it's a wonderful core-strengthening pose as the abdominal muscles have to work hard to round the back while maintaining the partner's weight. This is a very stable pose with the weight being supported by four limbs and the body being in close proximity to the ground.

Symbolism: The symbolism in Cat/Cow with a Starfish is that sometimes one partner has to do more of the work while the other rests, but that there's a balance because soon the roles are reversed, so the work and rest are evenly divided in this pose.

This pose is a variation on Cat/Cow *(Bidalasana/Marjaryasana).*

Upright Back Chair

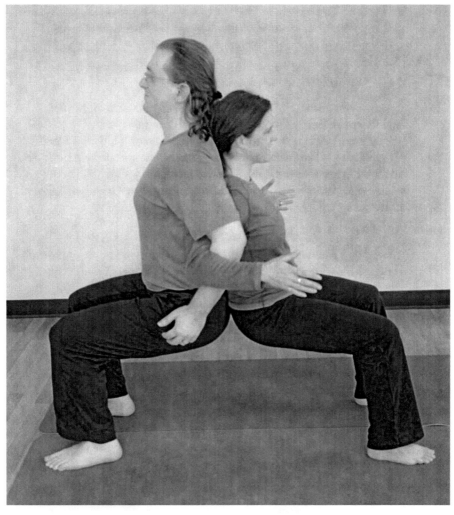

1. Begin with both partners standing back-to-back.

2. Partners hook their elbows together.

3. Keeping their backs together by engaging through the abdominals, both partners begin to walk the feet forward away from their partner.

4. Partners keep their own feet just slightly wider than hip-width apart and both the heel and kneecap lined up with the second toe.

5. When the knees come down to a 90-degree angle, with the thighs parallel to the floor, partners hold this pose for four complete breath cycles.

    •   Make sure neither partner holds the pose below 90-degrees, as that will strain the knee joint.

    •   If it is difficult for either partner to drop down to a 90-degree angle with their knees, both partners can hold the pose at a higher level.

Upright Back Chair builds tremendous strength in the quadriceps muscle group of the thighs. It's reminiscent of wall sits, which many sports conditioning programs use to build leg strength. Upright Back Chair also establishes solid alignment in the hips, knees, and ankles to maintain a good kinetic chain in the legs. By keeping the backs together, partners learn to use core muscles to maintain good posture.

Symbolism: The symbolism in Upright Back Chair is that even though you cannot see each other in this pose, you know you are still connected and can feel the strength of your partner. Your partner literally has "got your back."

This pose is a variation on Chair *(Utkatasana)*.

Armchair

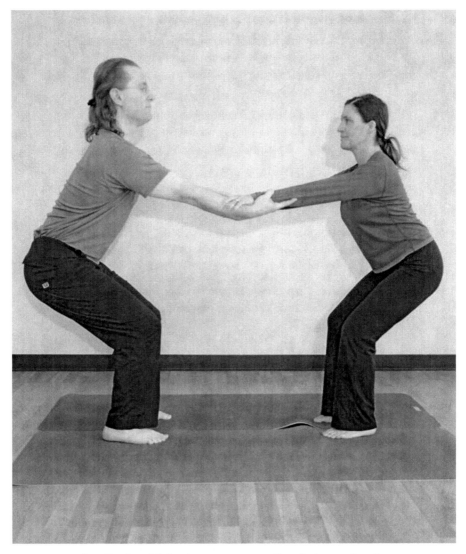

1. Begin with both partners standing facing each other, a few inches apart.

2. Both partners grab each others' forearms firmly but without digging in with fingernails.

   - Partners should roll up sleeves if either of them has trouble establishing a firm grasp on fabric-covered forearms.

3. Both partners walk backwards away from their partner, bending their knees and folding at the hip crease, keeping their own feet hip-width apart and making sure that the kneecap points towards the second toe.

   - If the heights are dramatically different, the taller partner may take his feet slightly wider, still making sure that the kneecap points towards the second toe.

4. Partners keep the chests lifted and the abdominal muscles strongly drawing inward, so that the lower back stays long in this pose.

5. Tailbones reach back and down, as if the partners were about to sit into a chair, bending at the hip crease.

6. The weight should be in the heels of the feet, and the toes should feel light; partners can lift their toes in this pose to make sure the weight is in their heels.

7. Partners keep the shoulders pulling down away from the ears and the shoulders pulling back into their sockets.

8. When the knees come almost to a 90-degree angle, both partners stop and hold the pose for four complete breath cycles.

Similar to the Upright Back Chair pose, Armchair builds great strength in the quadriceps and hamstrings in the legs. This pose also develops great strength in the gluteus muscles of the hips. It also develops strength in the adductors (inner thigh) and abductors (outer thigh) that serve as stabilizers in this pose. By asking the partners to maintain an upright position for the chest, Armchair builds strength in the back. Armchair also uses slightly more abdominal strength than in Upright Back Chair to prevent the lower back from overarching.

Symbolism: The symbolism of this Armchair is the inter-dependency between the partners. If one partner lets go, the other would probably stumble. This emphasizes how it takes two people contributing what they can to form a solid relationship.

This pose is a variation on Chair *(Utkatasana)*.

Extended Table

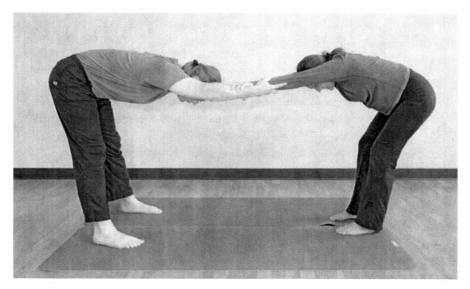

1. Begin with both partners standing facing each other.

2. Both partners hold each others' forearms without leaving deep impressions on the skin.

3. Both partners walk backwards away from their partner with relatively straight legs, keeping their own feet hip-width apart.

4. Knees can have a soft bend to them; note that if the heights are dramatically different, the taller partner will have to bend his knees more and may even take his feet slightly wider than hip-width apart.

5. Partners reach their tailbones back and the crown of the head forward, folding at the hips instead of the waist.

6. Ears come between the upper arms, keeping the head in line with the spine.

7. When the backs come roughly parallel to the floor, both partners stop and hold the pose for four complete breath cycles.

Extended Table lengthens the spine, providing gentle traction to elongate the erector spinae in the back. Extended Table is wonderful for creating space back after it has been compressed while seated for a long time—such as when we sit at a desk all day—making this a great end-of-the-workday pose. You will also notice a decent opening in the hamstrings along the back of the legs as you practice Extended Table.

By reaching for your partner's arms, you create length in the latissimus dorsi, a large muscle group in the outside middle of your back. It also helps stretch the tissues of the armpits and the rib cage.

Symbolism: The symbolism of Extended Table is the growth that happens when two people work together towards the same goal.

This pose is a variation on Half Forward Fold (*Ardha Uttanasana*).

Two Warriors

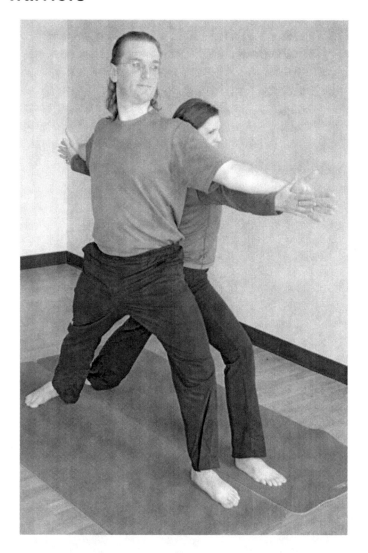

1. Begin with both partners standing back-to-back; there can be a small gap between their backs.

2. Both partners take the feet out wide; stretching the arms straight out to the sides, the ankles should line up just below the wrists.

3. Partners intertwine arms like a twisted licorice stick, keeping extension from the shoulder through the fingertips.

4. Partner A turns both sets of toes to her right, with her right foot forming a 90-degree angle to her torso and the left foot turning slightly to the right.

5. Partner B turns both sets of toes to his left, with his left foot forming a 90-degree angle to his torso and the right foot turning slightly to the left.

6. Partner A bends her right knee, coming down to a 90-degree angle and keeping the left knee straight as Partner B bends his left knee, coming down to a 90-degree angle and keeping the right knee straight.

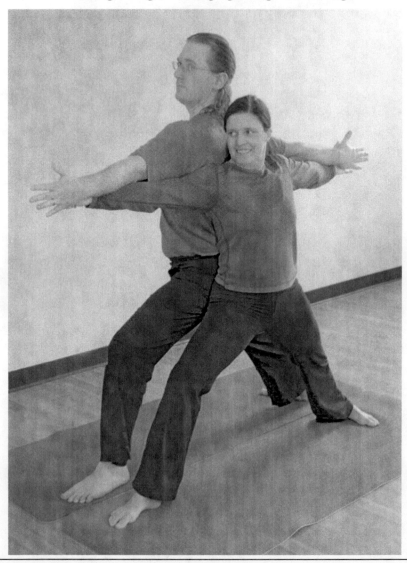

7. The bent knees should line up straight over the ankle, with the bent knee pointing towards the second toe; on the bent knee side, only the big toe should be visible when gazing down at the forward foot.

8. Partners keep the chest over the hips and the abdominal muscles engaged so the lower back lengthens instead of arching; partners can view this as drawing their hips forward, away from their partner.

9. Both partners extend the arms strongly, all the way through the fingertips, and keep the shoulders broad and the chest open.

10. Partner A looks to her right and Partner B to his left with focus, holding for four complete breath cycles.

From here, instead of switching sides immediately, you can go into Double Angle and then Just Right Triangle on this side first. Then you switch sides by pointing your feet to the opposite direction. You also can change the intertwine of your arms when you switch sides.

Two Warriors helps open the hips by opening the adductor muscles of the inner thighs. Like most other standing poses, it strengthens both the quadriceps and hamstring muscles of the thighs. It also builds strength in the back and outside of the hips. With the arms intertwined, this pose also becomes a great chest opener.

Symbolism: The symbolism in Two Warriors is the concept of both partners fighting on the same side rather than on opposite sides as they advance forward as one unit.

This pose is a variation on Warrior 2 *(Virabhadrasana 2).*

Double Angle

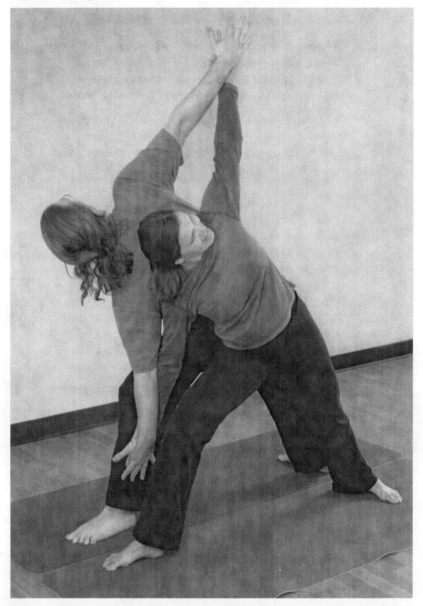

1. Begin from Two Warriors pose.

2. Keeping the front knees bent, back legs straight, and the arms intertwined, Partner A drops her chest down toward her right thigh while Partner B drops his chest down toward his left thigh.

3. Though the chest reaches down towards the thighs, the torso does not rest on the thigh; instead, partners engage their oblique muscles along the outside of their abdomen to support the torso.

4. Both partners let their bottom arms fall in between their knees as the top arm reaches up to the sky, keeping a bit of space between the shoulders and the ears.

5. After establishing the arms, both partners check to see that the bent knee is still lined up directly over the ankle.

6. Arches of the feet stay lifted as Partner A extends through the outside edge of her left foot and Partner B extends through the outside edge of his right foot.

7. Both partners look up to the sky if that is easy for the neck, otherwise they can face out, or even down towards the ground.

8. Partners hold the pose for four complete breath cycles.

Instead of coming up and moving on to the other side, you can go into Just Right Triangle on this side first, then switch sides and start with Two Warriors on the other side.

Double Angle continues the opening of the hips initiated by Two Warriors, while adding in a great side opener. It also helps open the muscles of the torso, particularly the quadratus lumborum in the back.

Symbolism: The symbolism of Double Angle is in the arms—while one arm is reaching down the other arm is reaching up, symbolizing how a great partner can help ground you while also lifting you up.

This pose is a variation on Extended Angle *(Utthita Parsvakonasana).*

Just Right Triangle

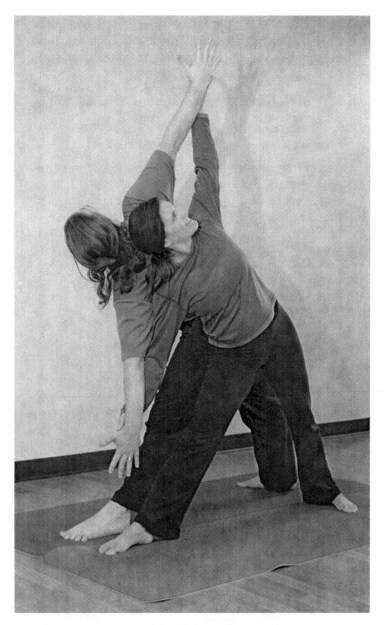

1. Begin from Double Angle pose.

2. Both Partners lift their chests about an inch higher and straighten their bent knee by strongly contracting the quadriceps in the front of the thigh.

3. Partner A extends out through the right armpit and Partner B through the left armpit, as both partners stretch through the ribs, keeping both sides of the rib cage long, not rounded.

4. Partner A reaches her right hand down towards her right shin as Partner B reaches his left hand down towards his left shin.

5. Partners reach the top arms towards the sky.

6. Partners keep the arches of the feet lifted and the quadriceps of the thighs strongly engaged.

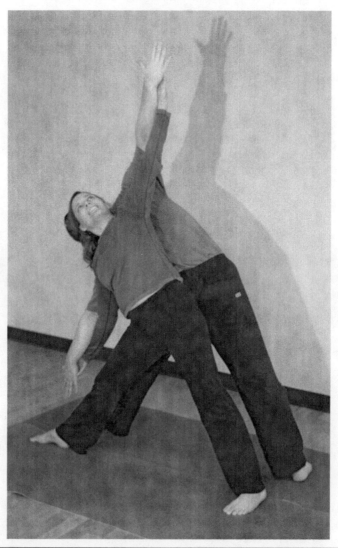

7. Partner A can have a slight bend in her front knee (her right knee) and Partner B can have a slight bend in his front knee (his left knee), but the back knees stay straight in this pose.

8. Partners can turn their heads to look up in this pose, or just find any comfortable position for the neck; partners can also practice a rotation exercise for the neck by turning to look up with each inhale and down with each exhale.

9. Hold this pose for four complete breath cycles.

After Just Right Triangle, you can switch sides and repeat the Two Warriors, Double Angle, Just Right Triangle sequence on the other side.

Just Right Triangle has the same side-torso-extending benefits as Double Angle, but it adds a good stretch for the hamstrings on the back of the thigh. On this side, Partner A feels a hamstring stretch in the back of her right thigh, while Partner B feels it in his left thigh. By extending the hands all the way through the fingertips, it helps undo some of the constant bending of the knuckles most people do while at the keyboard all day.

Symbolism: The symbolism of Just Right Triangle is in the angles created. Angles are the convergence of two lines, such as when the two lives of the partners finally converge and create this great geometry.

This pose is a variation on Triangle *(Trikonasana).*

Super Straddle

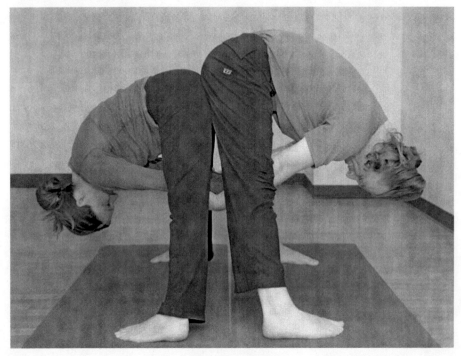

1. Begin with both partners standing back-to-back with a few inches of space between them.

2. Both partners stretch their arms straight out to the side, then step their feet as wide as their hands so that their ankles line up approximately under their wrists.

   • Taking a narrower stance makes it a harder stretch, while moving the feet further apart makes it an easier pose.

3. Both partners turn their toes inward and heels outward, so their feet are slightly pigeon-toed.

4. Both partners bring their hands to their hips.

5. Keeping the legs very straight and strong, and engaging the abdominal muscles, both partners fold forward from the hips, reaching their back long instead of rounding.

   • Unlike some poses where bending the knees modifies the pose to protect the back, the angle of the knees in this pose requires partners to keep the knees straight; bending the knees would cause an uncomfortable alignment.

6. Once they are down as far as they can go, partners reach between their legs to grab their partner's arms and work their chests towards each other.

7. Partners allow the neck to fully relax in this pose and for the head to just hang as they hold for four complete breath cycles.

Super Straddle helps open the inner thighs and hamstrings in the backs of the thighs. The gentle pull from the partner helps further stretch the lower back. Because this is a forward fold, it can have a calming effect on the brain. It also provides traction on the neck, relieving some tension that can accumulate in the cervical spine.

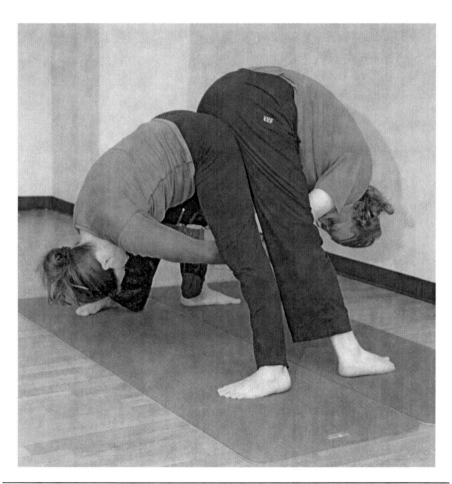

If one partner has difficulty reaching between the legs, place a chair in front of her and have her rest her arms on the chair while the other partner reaches for the legs of the chair.

Symbolism: The symbolism in Super Straddle is remembering how much work it takes to get close to someone, which helps you value your relationships even more.

This pose is a variation on Standing Straddle *(Prasarita Padotttanasana).*

Double Down Dog

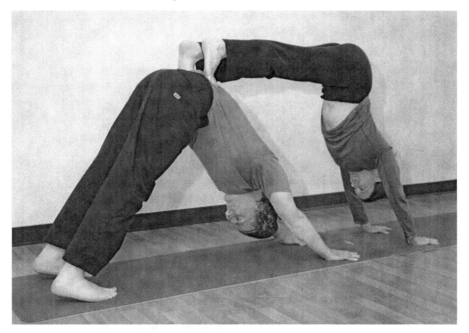

1. Partner B begins by taking his hands and knees onto the floor.

2. Partner B keeps his fingers spread wide and middle finger pointing forward.

3. Partner B walks his knees back several inches behind his hips.

4. Curling the toes on the floor, Partner B lifts his hips high up in the air and presses his hips back.

5. Keeping the knees slightly bent, Partner B presses his heels toward the floor.

6. Partner B lets his ears hang between his upper arms, and spreads the shoulders away from the spine, coming into a solo Downward Facing Dog pose.

7. Once Partner B has established his pose, Partner A stands in between Partner B's hands.

8. Partner A folds forward, bending her knees and taking her palms to the floor one to two feet in front of Partner B's hands, depending on Partner A's height.

9.   Partner A keeps her fingers spread wide and middle finger pointing forward.

10. Partner A lifts one foot, then the other, taking both feet onto Partner B's back.

     •   An option for Partner A, if she does not want to put her feet on Partner B's back, is just to take her own Downward-Facing Dog pose in front of her partner.

     •   Another option is to just provide an assist to Partner B by standing behind him and gently pulling his thighs back.

     •   A third option is to just take one foot at a time onto Partner B's back, hold for four breath cycles, then change feet, as if doing a Three-Legged Dog.

11. Partner A walks her feet as close to Partner B's hip bones as possible, possibly resting her heels on Partner B's hip bones.

12. Partners hold for four complete breath cycles.

13. To come out of this pose, Partner A gently hops down, straddling Partner B's hands, and bending her knees for a soft landing.

Double Down Dog has numerous benefits. For Partner B, the backward pressure of Partner A's feet helps him achieve more length in the spine, providing a greater stretch in the erector spinae muscles of the back. Partner B will feel his hands become lighter on the floor, and may even someday get to take them off the floor. This is also a great calf stretch for Partner B. For Partner A, this is almost a Half Handstand, making it a wonderful strengthener for her upper body, particularly the triceps muscles in her arms.

Symbolism: The symbolism of Double Down Dog is that if your partner provides a solid base, you can take a risk and really amaze yourself and maybe even take flight.

This pose is a variation on Downward Facing Dog (*Adho Mukha Svanasana*).

Open Hearted Warrior

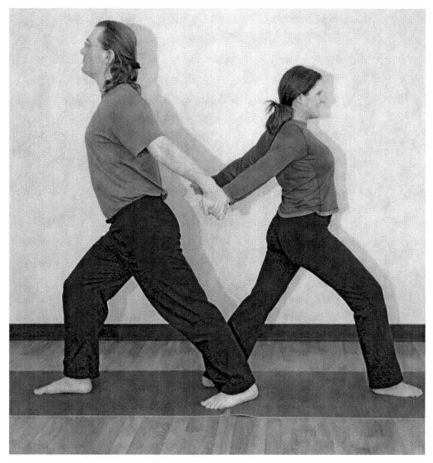

1. Begin with Partner A and Partner B standing, facing away from each other.

2. Both partners step their right foot forward two feet, staggering their back feet so their left feet are in line with each other, but a few inches apart.

3. The left feet should be angled so that the toes point to roughly eleven o'clock.

4. Each partner should line their front heel up roughly with the arch of their back foot.

5. Keeping their hips squared towards their front leg, both partners bend their front knees, keeping their back legs straight, coming in to Warrior 1 pose.

6. Both partners keep their abdominal muscles and gluteus muscles strong, pulling their hips forward and pointing their tailbone down to avoid overarching the lower back and to create a greater opening in the hip flexors on the back leg.

7. Both partners reach their hands back and clasp their partner's hands.

8. Using the security of the hand clasp, both partners extend their chests forward away from each other to create a great chest opener.

9. Hold this pose for four breath cycles before switching feet.

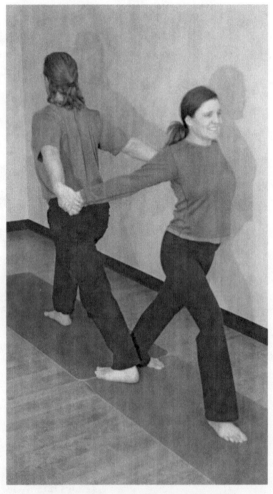

Open Hearted Warrior is a strong chest opener. It stretches the pectoral muscles in the chest and the anterior deltoid in the shoulder. With our daily work activities, such as working at a computer, these muscles stay contracted throughout the day and get really tight, making chest openers very important to maintain balance in the body. This pose also stretches the hip flexors that get very tight with the amount of sitting most of us do throughout the day, which keeps the hip flexors in constant state of contraction. Hip flexors also give us power for activities such as hiking and biking, but they can cause lower back pain if they are too tight.

Symbolism: The symbolism of Open Hearted Warrior comes from the dichotomy inherent in the name. We often think of warriors as angry, but if we consider the term warrior in a broader sense, as someone who fights for justice and against oppression, then this pose is a tribute to those warriors. When practicing with a partner, this pose symbolizes the courage it takes to open your heart, which can be scarier than fighting even the toughest opponent.

This pose is a variation on Warrior 1 *(Virabhadrasana 1).*

Double Cobra

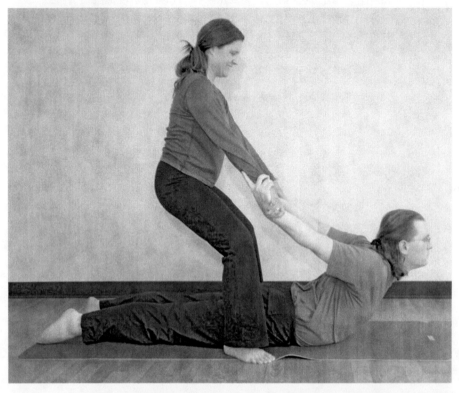

1. Begin with Partner B lying face down on the ground.

2. Partner A stays standing, straddling Partner B with her feet lined up roughly near Partner B's hips.

3. Partner A bends her knees into a squat, bending at the hips and the knees; the knees point towards the second toe.

4. Partner A reaches down to grab Partner B's arms as Partner B reaches his arms back to reach Partner A's arms.

5. Both partners grab forearms or hands solidly but without causing pain.

6. Partner B keeps his feet pressing firmly into the floor, with the gluteus muscles in the back of the hip and quadriceps muscles in the fronts of the thighs strongly engaged.

7. Partner B keeps his abdominal muscles engaged to support the lower back and ground the tailbone.

8. Keeping her back straight, and lifting with the legs, Partner A begins to lift Partner B's chest off the ground, stopping when Partner B says he has reached his limit.

9. Partner A can keep her knees slightly bent and take a standing backbend to open the front of her body, or she can stay in a squat and just work on leg strength.

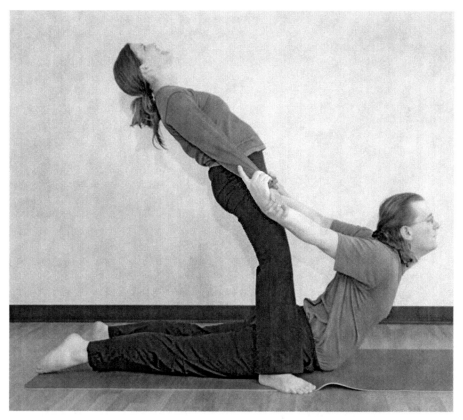

10. After holding for four complete breath cycles, Partner A bends her knees to lower Partner B to the floor.

11. Since this is a big back bend, Partner B should rest on the floor with his head resting on folded forearms to neutralize the spine for four complete breath cycles before switching positions.

Double Cobra is also a huge chest opener, opening up tight pectoralis muscles and the anterior deltoids in the front of the shoulder; it also helps extend the rectus abdominus muscles in the abdomen region It's a deeper backbend than the Open Hearted Warrior pose, so you should ease your way into and out of this pose.

Symbolism: The symbolism in Double Cobra is in the communication. By telling your partner when you have had enough, this pose is an excellent exercise in setting boundaries positively, and in respecting your partner's boundaries.

This pose is a variation on Cobra *(Bhujangasana)*.

Twister Triangle

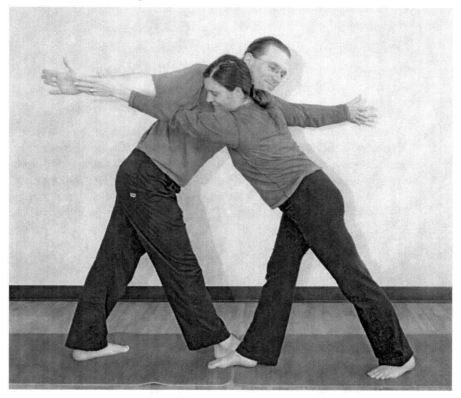

1. Begin with both partners standing facing each other, roughly two feet apart.

2. Both partners step their right foot forward so that the outside edges of both partners' forward feet touch.

3. Both partners turn their back toes out a bit; the front heel should point to the middle of the back foot.

    *   The further away the back foot is, the harder this pose becomes.

4. Both partners square their hips forward to face each other.

5. The knees stay as straight as possible; the front knee can have a slight bend but the back knee should stay straight.

6. Both partners hinge forward at the hips, keeping the back straight.

7. Holding the forward reach and a long straight back, both partners twist to face each other coming into a Revolved Triangle pose.

8. Both partners reach their left hand forward to touch their partner's right arm, while reaching their right hand back to touch their partner's left arm.

9. After holding for four complete breath cycles breaths, partners switch feet to take the pose on the other leg.

Twister Triangle is complicated because it involves hamstring flexibility, hip flexibility, and rotation in the spine. This pose helps open the hamstring muscles in the back of the thigh, particularly in the front leg, and helps open the gastrocnemius and soleus muscles in the calves

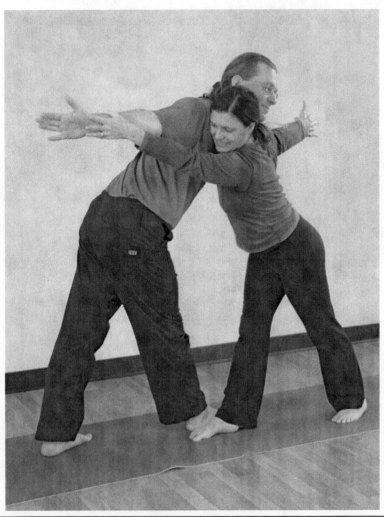

and ankles, particularly on the back leg. It also helps open some deep lower back and hip muscles, such as the piriformus.

While Twister Triangle can be tricky to get into the first several times you practice, it actually helps you maintain better form than by practicing Revolved Triangle by yourself. Having the support of your partner rather than reaching your forward hand to the floor allows you to keep more length in the spine and avoid rounding the back.

Symbolism: The symbolism of Twister Triangle is that by asking for help we can make ourselves stronger. By using a partner for extra stability and balance, you keep more integrity in the pose than when you try to balance with your forward arm on your forward leg. This teaches us that getting a little help from our friends makes us better.

This pose is a variation on Revolved Triangle *(Pavritta Trikonasana).*

Warrior 6 (Warrior 3 x 2)

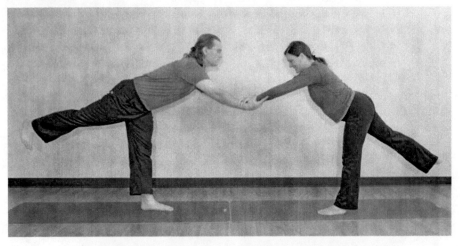

1. Begin with both partners standing facing each other, coming first into the Extended Table pose to determine how far apart to stand.

2. Both partners grab hands or forearms firmly.

3. Stabilizing their left legs and keeping the left knee straight, both partners reach their right toes a few inches behind the left leg while keeping the toes on the floor.

4. Simultaneously, both partners lift the right foot off the floor.

5. The right foot stays flexed, as partners extend back through the heels and point the toes straight down towards the floor.

6. The quadriceps muscles on both the left and the right thighs stay strongly engaged.

7. For every inch the right foot rises, lower the chest the same amount, with the torso coming no further down than parallel to the floor and the right leg coming no higher than hip level.

   • Partners can bend forward different amounts from each other.

8. Both partners engage abdominals to keep the spine neutral and the hips level; the right hip may want to pop up, but keeping it level makes the balance easier.

9. After holding for four complete breath cycles, partners switch feet to take the pose on the other leg.

Warrior 6 is a great balance pose that also helps stretch the hamstrings in the back of the thighs and elongates the spine. It also demonstrates the concept of neutral spine, because when the back either arches or rounds in this pose, it makes the balance more difficult.

Whereas working with a partner makes some poses harder, it often makes Warrior 6 an easier pose for people. The big challenge in working with a partner here is that people have varying degrees of flexibility in their hamstrings, and this might mean not coming into your full range on this pose. This teaches you a great lesson to enjoy your yoga practice wherever you land in each pose.

Symbolism: The symbolism of Warrior 6 is that the seesaw-like action of the leg rising and chest descending in this pose demonstrates the balancing act of a relationship. For every movement, there is a counter movement, just like in a relationship that for every give there is an equal take.

This pose is a variation on Warrior 3 *(Virabhadrasana 3)*.

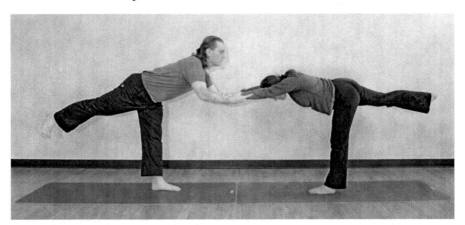

Gibbous Moon

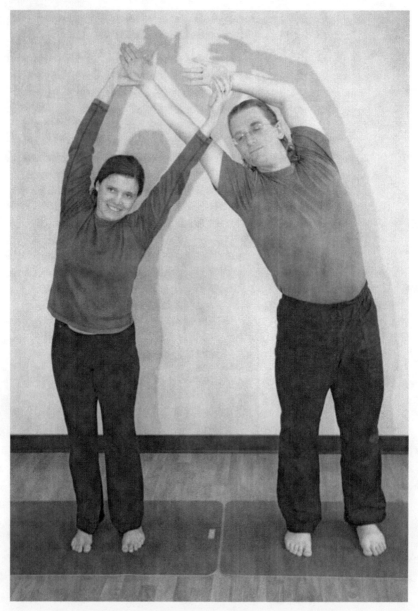

1. Begin with both partners standing side-by-side, roughly two feet apart.

2. Both partners keep their own feet hip-width apart, legs strong and straight.

3. To keep the lower back long, both partners keep the abdominal muscles engaged and the tailbone pointed down.

4. Both partners reach their arms up overhead and into the center.

5. With her left hand, Partner A embraces Partner B's left hand, and with his right hand, Partner B joins Partner A's right hand.

6. While this pose will curve the spine to the side, the emphasis is on extending and reaching, rather than curving.

7. Hold this pose for four complete breath cycles.

Instead of switching sides right away, you can stay here and go directly into Long Neck on this side.

Gibbous Moon helps open the sides of the body, including the serratus anterior muscles along the rib cage. By opening these muscles, you create more room for the breath in your torso. This pose also moves the spine from side-to-side, providing great nourishment to the joints of the spine.

Symbolism: The symbolism in Gibbous Moon is the completeness of the shape. By doing this pose solo you create a crescent moon or a half moon shape, but by adding a partner, you create a fuller gibbous moon, in the same way that our friends and loved ones fill our lives with joy.

This pose is a variation on Standing Side Bend, also known as Half Moon *(Ardha Chandrasana)*.

Long Neck

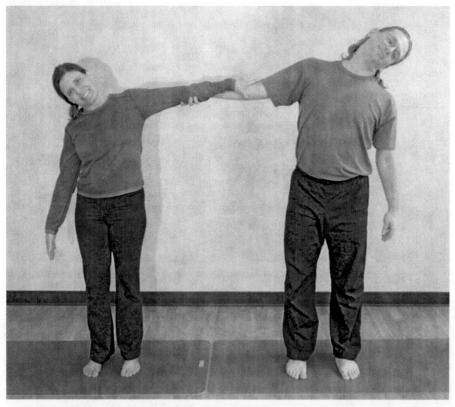

1. Begin with both partners standing side-by-side in Gibbous Moon.

2. Both partners step an additional foot away from their partner.

3. Using the inside arms, both partners hold each other's forearms.

4. Keeping the legs and the body straight, the abdominals and quadriceps work to align the body.

5. Both partners lean their outside ear towards their outside shoulder, reaching their head away from their partner.

6. Partners should feel some dynamic tension as they both pull away.

7. Both partners keep their shoulders dropping down away from their ears.

8. After holding for four breath cycles, switch sides and begin with Gibbous Moon.

Long Neck helps open some muscles in the neck and shoulder region, such as the levator scapulae and the upper trapezius. These muscles tend to hold a lot of tension, particularly for people who shrug their shoulders up during the day. This pose helps create length in the neck and shoulder while relieving some accumulated tension.

Symbolism: The symbolism of Long Neck is merely to open up and release tension in places where tension often accumulates. When you can stop holding the body in a constant state of vigilance, and learn to relax, you can open up more to the people you care about.

This pose is derived from stretches we have learned from physical therapists.

Double Tree

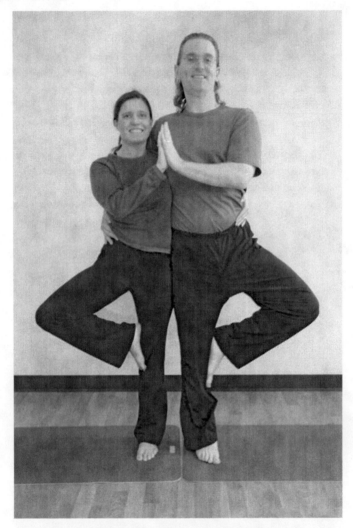

1. Begin with both partners standing side-by-side, hips touching, inside feet roughly six inches apart.

2. Both partners keep their own feet hip-width apart, with the legs strong and straight.

3. To keep the lower back in neutral alignment, partners draw their abdominal muscles inward.

4. Reaching around the partner's lower back with the inside arm, both partners grab each other's hips gently.

5. Both partners take their outside hands towards the center, pressing their palm against their partner's palm.

6. Partner A comes onto the toes of her outside foot, bending her outside knee and turning it out to the side.

7. Partner A draws her outside foot either below or above her inside knee, without pressing the heel directly into the knee; the outside foot presses firmly into the standing leg while the standing leg presses firmly into the outside foot, creating dynamic tension.

   • An option is to keep the outside toes on the floor for extra stability.

   • For additional stability, partners can practice facing a wall, and brace the outside hand against the wall for balance.

8. After Partner A has stabilized in her Tree, Partner B goes into his Tree, following the same procedure.

9. The hips should stay more or less level in this pose; often this means making sure the outside hip stays level and does not pop up.

10. After holding the balance for four complete breath cycles, both partners switch sides to repeat.

Balance poses, such as Double Tree, help us focus the mind. You can't think about other things such as doing laundry or finishing a work proposal while holding a balance pose, so balance poses help de-clutter our mind—this has a calming effect on the body.

Double Tree is also a hip opening pose, stretching the inside of the hip and the adductor muscles of the inner thigh. This pose takes some negotiation with the foot position; you might find stepping the inside feet a bit further apart helps. It's also completely acceptable to try this pose several times with the outside toes on the floor. Ultimately you do want to keep the inside hip lining up over the ankle, so you do need to stand fairly close. One trick on getting into this pose is to have the person with the stronger sense of balance come into the pose first.

Symbolism: The symbolism of Double Tree is the subtlety of non-verbal communication and the adjustments you can make simply by sensing the balance or imbalance of your partner.

This pose is a variation on Tree *(Vrkasana)*.

Pas de Deux

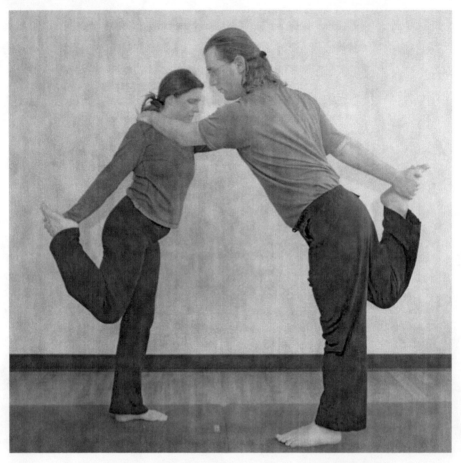

1. Begin with both partners standing facing each other, roughly two feet apart.

2. Partners stand slightly staggered so that Partner B's right foot lines up with Partner A's right foot.

3. Partners place their left hand on their partner's right shoulder for initial stability.

4. Partner A holds Partner B stable as Partner B bends his right knee, lifting his right foot towards the back of his right hip.

5. Partner B grabs his right foot with his right hand, grabbing the foot from the inside to avoid twisting the wrist.

   • If the right foot is not easily in reach, Partner B can wrap a necktie around the ball of his foot and hold the necktie in his right hand.

6. Once Partner B is stable, Partner A bends her right knee, lifting her right foot and taking her right foot into her right hand, using the same technique as Partner B.

7. Partner B then bends forward at the hip and reaches with his left hand to touch Partner A's right foot.

8. After Partner B is stable, Partner A bends forward at the hip and reaches with her left hand to touch Partner B's right foot.

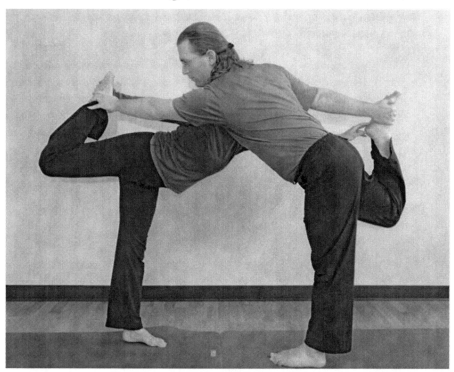

9. Keeping the right knees pointed directly to the floor, both partners kick into their right hand using the strength of the gluteus muscles, raising the right foot towards the sky.

10. As each partner's foot rises, both partners begin to fold forward at the hips; for every inch that the foot rises, the chest lowers in an equal amount.

   - An option for this pose is to try the Dancer pose solo, with Partner A standing firm like a mountain and Partner B practicing Dancer, leaning the front hand on Partner A for support.

11. After holding for four complete breath cycles, change sides to repeat on the other leg, remembering to change the stagger of the feet.

While some partner poses make the pose easier, this version of Dancer makes a difficult pose even more challenging. Pas de Deux is still a great leg and hip opening pose—it stretches the hip flexors in the hips and the quadriceps in the thighs. It also helps open the pectoral muscles in the chest and anterior deltoid in the shoulder by extending the back arm back to reach the foot. The stronger you kick up with your back leg, the more Pas de Deux becomes a great strengthener for the gluteus muscles in the back of the hip.

Symbolism: The symbolism in Pas de Deux is that learning to dance on your own is challenging, but learning to dance with a partner is even more challenging. This challenge, however, fuels tremendous growth and confidence.

This pose is a variation on Dancer *(Natarajasana)*.

Two Sided Plank

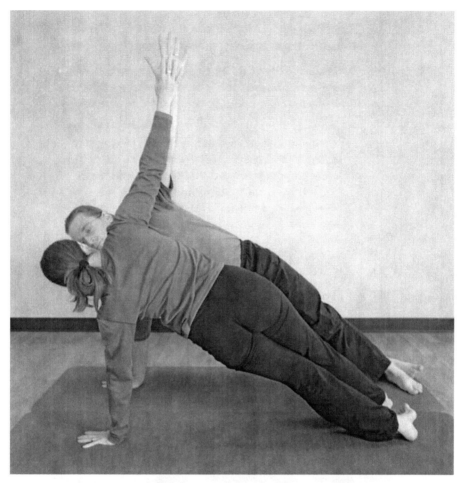

1. Begin with both partners on hands and knees side-by-side with Partner A's right hand next to Partner B's left hand; knees should be several inches behind the hips.

2. Both partners line up their the hands directly under the shoulders, fingers spread wide and middle finger pointing forward.

3. Engaging the abdominals and gluteus muscles for stability, both partners stretch their legs straight back, pressing their toes into the floor, coming into a side-by-side Plank.

4. The quadriceps in the thighs stay strong as the partners extend back through their heels and keep the hips lifted.

5. The triceps stay strong to keep the torso lifted in a strong neutral alignment without locking the elbow.

6. Partner A rolls onto the outside edge of her left foot, placing her right foot on the floor next to the left foot while reaching her right arm straight to the sky.

   • An option is to keep the left knee on the ground, swinging the left foot out to the side so the shin extends 90 degrees away from center (as if engaging the kickstand of a bicycle), and resting the left shin and foot on the floor while keeping the right leg straight.

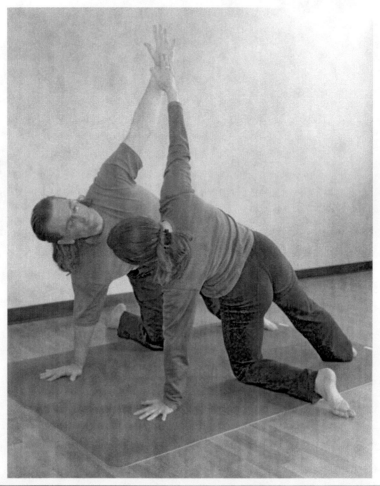

7. Partner B mirrors Partner A, rolling onto the outside edge of his right foot, placing his left foot on the floor next to his right foot, and reaching his left arm straight to the sky.

8. Once both partners have established their base, they can press their top hands into each other, extending their joined top hands skyward.

9. After four complete breath cycles, partners come back to an all fours position, then change sides.

Two Sided Plank is a great core strengthener and upper body strengthener. The muscles of the triceps in the upper arms work actively to keep the body up. The pectoral muscles in the chest and shoulder work, as do the muscles of the upper back. This pose also engages strongly through the core and the quadriceps to keep the hips lifted.

Two Sided Plank is a strong arm-balancing pose, but if you find pain in your wrists, then definitely modify the pose by coming onto your bottom knee, rather than having both legs straight.

Symbolism: The symbolism in Two Sided Plank is strength. Even when things start to go sideways, you can always draw strength from your relationships.

This pose is a variation on Side Plank *(Vasisthasana).*

Two Masted Boat

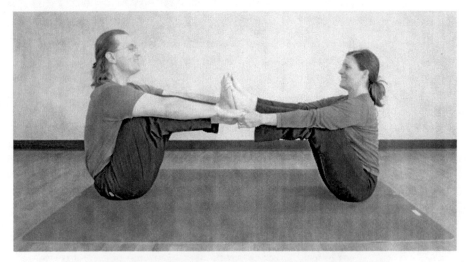

1. Begin with both partners sitting down facing each other with the knees bent and feet flat on the floor.

2. Partners should be close enough so their toes touch.

3. Partners join hands, keeping the shoulders drawing back into a neutral alignment.

4. Partner A presses the right foot into Partner B's left foot, bringing the feet up toward the sky; then the partners do the same with the other feet.

5. Keeping contact with the feet, partners keep their hands together.

   • An option is to take the hands out to the side; with this option, it is often easier to begin sitting further apart and not join hands at the beginning.

6. Both partners should find balance on their sacrum, the flat part of the spine just above their tailbone; they should not feel any sharp pressure on the tailbone.

7. The spine stays lifted and tall in this pose, just like the mast of a sailboat.

8. The knees can stay slightly bent, or completely straighten as the feet lift, as long as both partners can keep their backs long.

9. The neck and jaw should stay relaxed.

10. After holding for four complete breath cycles, partners can come out and rest, and then try this pose again; it is useful to practice this pose twice in a row.

Two Masted Boat strengthens the rectus abdominus muscles strongly. The challenging component of this pose is that the abdominal muscles work very hard while holding their length. Typically, when doing stomach crunches you contract, or shorten the rectus abdominus, but here we are asking the muscles to work just as hard while holding their length, or while being stretched. The hip flexors also work strongly in this pose. The erector spinae muscles in the back also work to stabilize you in this pose and prevent your spine from rounding.

If you feel any pressure on the tailbone, tip yourself back slightly, so that you balance on the sacrum, which lies just above your tailbone.

Symbolism: The symbolism of Two Masted Boat comes from the action of the abdominal muscles being engaged. This pose demonstrates that you can be strong but flexible at the same time, which is key to maintaining healthy relationships.

This pose is a variation on Boat *(Navasana).*

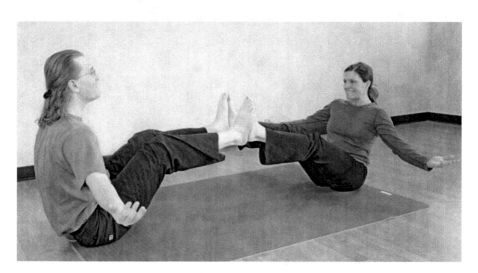

Diamond

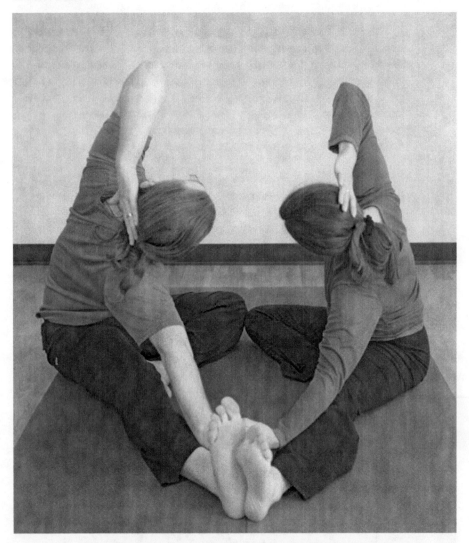

1. Both partners begin seated facing each other, coming knee-to-knee in a cross-legged sit.

2. Partner B stretches his right leg out to the side at approximately a 45-degree angle.

3. Partner B bends his left knee, taking his left foot into his right inner thigh, leaving some space between his left heel and the groin.

4. Partner A stretches her left leg out to the side at approximately a 45-degree angle.

5. Partner A bends her right knee, taking her right foot into her left inner thigh, leaving some space between her right heel and the groin.

6. Partner B reaches his right hand along his right leg, while Partner A reaches her left hand along her left leg.

7. Partner B's right hand grabs Partner A's left hand.

8. Both partners bring their free hand to the back of their heads and rotate the top elbow up and back to open the chest.

9. On the straight leg, the toes point towards the sky, flexing the foot and keeping the leg active.

10. Partner B reaches his right armpit down towards his right knee as Partner A reaches her left armpit down towards her left knee.

11. Both partners keep turning their chest up and away from each other, stretching long through the side.

   • An option for a partner with flexible hamstrings is to reach the top arm overhead and grab the toes of the straight leg; however, this should continue to be a straight side bend, without letting the chest turn downward.

12. After holding for eight complete breath cycles, partners change sides.

Diamond, like other side bends, helps to open the sides of the torso. This side bend helps open some muscles of the upper back, including the latissimus dorsi. Diamond also opens the hip on the bent leg and stretches the hamstring and calf on the straight leg.

Symbolism: The symbolism of Diamond is found in the movement of the heart away from the partner while the hands maintain contact. You stay connected while still feeling open and free. Great partnerships provide security without stifling.

This pose is a variation on Revolved Head to Knee *(Pavritta Janu Sirsasana)*.

Double Straddle

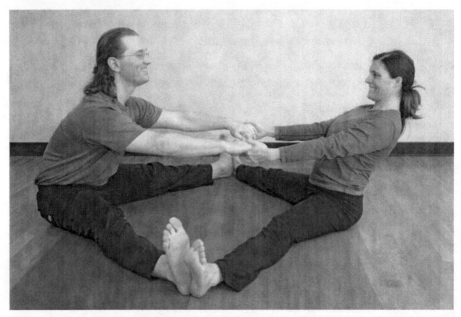

1. Begin with both partners seated with their legs stretched out wide and feet touching.

   - If flexibility in the hips and hamstrings prevents a partner from sitting up straight, elevate the hips by sitting on a folded mat or towel.

2. Toes stay pointed to the sky, with the feet flexed, and quadriceps muscles in the thighs engaged.

   - If a partner experiences any pain in the back of a knee, bending the knees is a safe modification.

3. Both partners grab hands or forearms.

4. With an inhaling breath, Partner A leans back as Partner B folds forward with an exhaling breath.

5. Both partners maintain length in their back using core strength.

6. After holding for eight complete breaths cycles, Partner B leans back as Partner A folds forward.

   - An option in this pose is to flow back and forth with the breath for a few times before holding the stretch.

Double Straddle has many benefits. For the partner folding forward, it helps open the hamstring muscles in the backs of the thighs and the adductor muscles in the inner things. In the forward fold, this pose also helps stretch the lower back. For the partner leaning back, this is an abdominal strengthener, similar to Two Masted Boat.

By flowing back and forth several times, you can practice Full Circle Breath, as the partner folding forward exhales, the partner leaning back exhales.

You definitely want to make this pose comfortable, and avoid compression in the lower back. Sitting on a folded mat or towel allows the pelvis to tip forward and the lower back to maintain its natural alignment.

Symbolism: The symbolism in Double Straddle is the process of surrendering. As one partner pulls backward, the partner folding forward learns to surrender and relax.

This pose is a variation on Seated Straddle *(Uphavista Konasana)*.

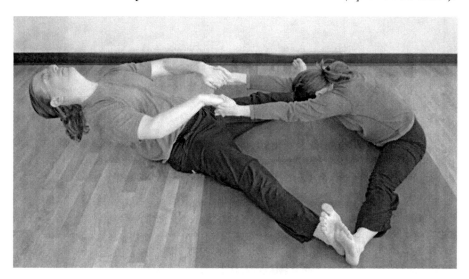

Forward Reach

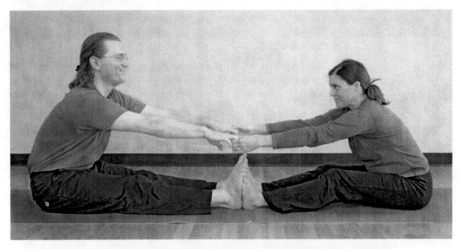

1. Both partners begin seated facing each other, legs stretched straight out in front; partners sit close enough so that they can press the soles of their feet into each other.

2. Keeping the spine long, both partners reach the chest forward.

    • Just like in Double Straddle, if the lower back rounds in this pose, elevate the hips by sitting on a folded mat or towel.

3. Staying strong in the fronts of the thighs without locking the knees, partners engage the quadriceps strongly; knees can have a slight bend to them.

4. Partners reach their hands towards the toes, maybe grabbing hands.

5. Shoulders draw back into their sockets.

6. When both partners have folded as far forward as they can, they can relax and round the spine.

7. Hold the pose for eight full breath cycles, then come up slowly.

Forward Reach is a huge stretch for the entire back of the legs—calves all the way through the hamstrings. It also stretches the lower back muscles, particularly the erector spinae.

Instead of rounding immediately, you should keep the spine as long as possible, then round for the last few moments. You can even elongate the time spent in this pose by holding with a straight back for eight full breath cycles, then relaxing and rounding for another eight full breath cycles.

Symbolism: The symbolism in Forward Reach is that by bowing forward you are honoring and giving thanks to your partner for the ways in which that person contributes to your health and happiness.

This pose is a variation on Seated Forward Fold *(Pashimottanasana).*

Proud Sit

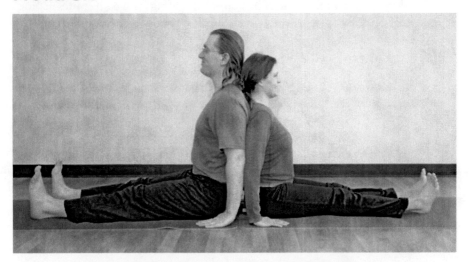

1. Begin with both partners sitting back to back with legs out straight in front; knees can bend slightly.

    *   Just like in Forward Reach, if the lower back rounds in this pose, elevate the hips by sitting on a folded mat or towel.

2. Hands rest on the floor next to the hips.

3. Arms stay strong, but the shoulders stay down away from the ears; if the shoulders hunch up, allow the elbows to bend more.

4. The thighs stay strong and the toes point straight up towards the sky.

5. Both partners sit up tall, engaging their abdominals and pressing into their partner's backs with a tall proud back.

6. Because the backs are together, partners can feel each other's inhalations and exhalations, which makes this an excellent pose to practice with Full Circle Breath.

7. Hold the pose for eight complete breath cycles.

After holding Proud Sit, you will probably want to relax and come into Open Cobbler's next.

Proud Sit is very simple, yet very strong. Classically, the solo version of this pose, Staff, is done to work on postural muscles. Using a partner makes this pose easier, and also allows us to hold it longer. The muscles of the rhomboids in the upper back, and even the abdominal muscles help us sit up tall. Proud Sit helps remind the body of correct posture.

Symbolism: The symbolism in Proud Sit is the deceptive simplicity of it. From the outside, it looks like you are just sitting doing nothing, when in fact your muscles are working hard to keep you sitting up tall. The same is true in relationships: they all take work and effort—even the ones that from an outside perspective appear to be effortless.

This pose is a variation on Staff *(Dandasana).*

Open Cobbler's

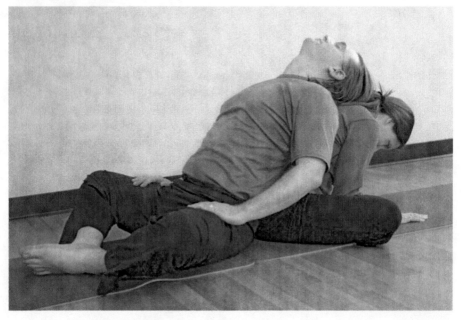

1. Begin from Proud Sit.

2. Bending the knees, both partners take the soles of their own feet together, letting the knees fall towards the floor.

3. Feet should be several inches away from the groin to allow some space in the back of the knee.

4. Partner A folds forward from the hips as Partner B reclines on Partner A's back.

5. Partner B can open up his arms and rest his hands wherever it allows his chest to open comfortably; he can rest his hands either on the floor, on his thighs, or on Partner A's knees.

6. After eight complete breath cycles, Partner B folds forward and Partner A reclines back to switch.

   - Another option is for partners to flow back and forth a few times before holding this pose, just like in Double Straddle; if they do flow, the partner reclining back inhales as the partner folding forward exhales.

Open Cobbler's is a great hip opener for the partner folding forward, opening the inner thighs. For the partner reclining back, along with opening the hips, Open Cobbler's provides a great opening in the chest. When you recline back, you release the pectoralis muscles in the chest.

Open Cobbler's is a very calming pose, which makes it a great pose to do before bedtime.

Symbolism: The symbolism in Open Cobbler's is that even though simultaneously both partners are opening up in different areas, the pose is still mutually beneficial. In a relationship, people do not always have to be doing the exact same thing to be mutually supportive and receive great benefit.

This pose is a variation on Cobbler's Pose, also known as Bound Angle *(Baddha Konasana)*.

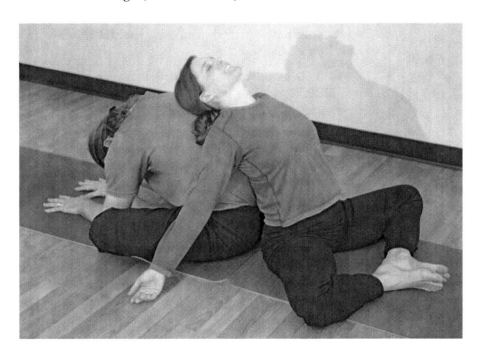

Child's Play

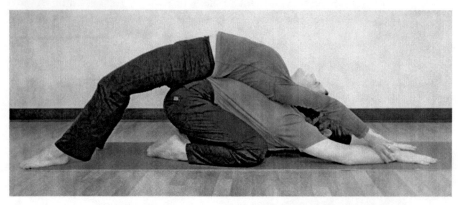

1. Begin with Partner B coming on to his knees, taking the big toes together and knees slightly wider than hip-width apart.

2. Partner B relaxes his torso onto his legs, stretching his hands forward on the floor.

3. Partner B places his forehead on the floor, coming into Child's Pose.

   - If the neck or back are uncomfortable with the face resting on the floor, an option is for Partner B to either cross his arms and rest his head on his forearms, or stack his fists on the floor and rest his forehead on his fists.

4. Once Partner B is settled, Partner A stands, facing away from Partner B, straddling Partner B's knees.

5. Partner A squats down, taking her hips on top of Partner B's hips.

6. Partner A supports herself by holding on to Partner B's hips, then reclines back.

   - Partner A checks in with Partner B to make sure he feels no uncomfortable pressure on his knees; if he does feel uncomfortable, Partner A can sit by his side instead, gently pressing his hips back with the palms of her hands.

7. After reclining, Partner A can stretch her arms overhead and her legs straight out in front of her.

8. After holding eight complete breath cycles, Partner A bends her knees into a squat, puts her hands on Partner B's hips, and uses the strength of her legs to stand up.

    - If Partner A has trouble coming up to standing, especially after being so low to the floor, Partner B can help by pushing up onto all fours, then tipping back to gently dump Partner A onto her feet; Partner A can also try slowly rolling off to the side, bracing with her hands and feet.

9. Before switching sides, Partner B should rest for a few moments in a solo Child's Pose.

For Partner B, Child's Play helps lengthen the muscles of the back, particularly the erector spinae. The weight of Partner A on his back helps deepen the stretch. For Partner A, this pose is another great backwards-bending pose, opening up the abdomen and the pectoralis muscles in the chest. If she extends her legs, Child's Play will also open the hip flexor muscles.

Symbolism: The symbolism in Child's Play is that learning to enjoy, trust, and surrender to the support of a partner can be quite blissful.

This pose is a variation on Child's Pose *(Balasana)*.

Double Twist

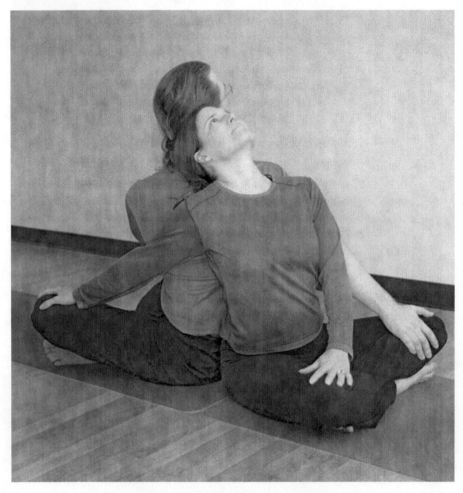

1. Begin with both partners sitting back to back in a cross-legged position.

2. Partners maintain a tall spine throughout this pose.

3. Both partners twist around to the right, resting their right hands on their partner's left knee; the left hand can rest on the floor or anywhere on their own legs.

4. Hips stay level on the ground.

   - One option is for the partners to also bring their heads back, resting the head either on their partner's head or shoulder, depending upon height differences.

5. For this pose, partners can breathe simultaneously, instead of using Full Circle Breath, by inhaling to sit up taller and exhaling to deepen the twist.

6. After holding for eight complete breaths, both partners unwind, change the cross of their legs, and twist to the left; the leg change is important so that both hips get an equal stretch.

Double Twist provides rotation in the spine. This pose both strengthens and opens the internal and external oblique muscles in the abdominal region: as you twist to one side, you open the other.

Like other twists, this helps relieve tension in the back. By rotating the spine slowly like this, you are moving synovial fluid between the discs of the spine, lubricating the joints and providing nourishment to the ligaments. Twists are also said to be stimulating for internal organs as they bring a deliberate compression that temporarily squeezes the blood supply, and when you release the pose, fresh blood and oxygen rush in.

The optional neck release helps unwind muscles of the neck and jaw, including the sternocleidomastoid. We tend to crane our necks forward constantly throughout the day while we stare at computer screens, work with our hands, or drive our cars; this makes opening the front of the neck, as you can in Double Twist, very important for balancing the muscles of the neck.

Symbolism: The symbolism of Double Twist is the graceful intertwining of lives that happen with solid relationships.

This pose is a variation on Seated Twist *(Bharadvajasana).*

Lords and Ladies of the Fishes

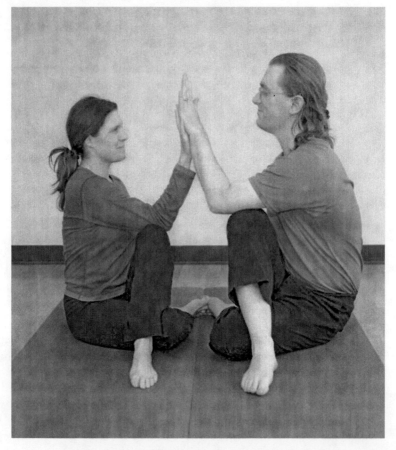

1. Begin with both partners sitting side-by-side with legs
   straight out in front, Partner B to the left of
   Partner A.

2. Partner B bends his right knee, crossing the right leg
   over the left and placing his right foot to the outside
   of his left knee; the right knee points upward.

3. Partner B bends his left knee, taking his left foot to the
   outside of his right hip.

4. Partner A bends her left knee, crossing the left leg
   over the right and placing her left foot to the outside
   of her right knee; the left knee points upward.

5. Partner A bends her right knee, taking her right foot
   to the outside of her left hip.

6. Both partners twist inward to face each other.

7. Partner B rests his right hand on the floor behind him as Partner A rests her left hand on the floor behind her.

8. Partner B puts his left hand in to center, placing his left elbow over his right knee.

   - Another option for Partner B is to take his left hand in to center, letting the left elbow rest on the inside of his right thigh, rather than coming over the knee.

9. Partner A takes her right hand in to center, drawing her right elbow over her left knee, and bringing her palm to touch Partner B's palm.

10. The shoulders stay relaxed and away from the ears.

11. The chest stays broad as the shoulder blades move out away from the spine.

12. The spine stays long and tall in this pose.

13. After holding for eight complete breath cycles, both partners unwind, then turn around to face the other direction and work on the other side.

Lords and Ladies of the Fishes is another great twist pose. This twist focuses more into the hip than Double Twist, stretching the gluteus maximus muscles in the back of the hip for the leg that crosses over the bottom leg. Lords and Ladies of the Fishes also opens the tensor fascia latae in the outer thigh and even some of the deep lower back muscles, such as the piriformis.

If you find the shoulders hunching forward and the chest caving in, try taking your elbow to the inside of your thigh rather than over the knee. If you find one hip pops up in this pose, you can take a folded mat or towel underneath that hip so your hips can relax.

Symbolism: The symbolism in Lords and Ladies of the Fishes is in facing your partner honestly. By truly facing someone openly, we can form stronger relationships in our lives.

This pose is variation on Lord of the Fishes *(Ardha Matsyendrasana).*

Drawbridge

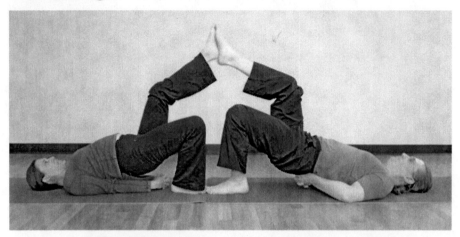

1. Begin with both partners sitting facing each other with knees bent, and feet flat on the floor, hip-width apart.

2. Partners should lie close enough so that their toes touch their partner's toes.

3. Both partners roll down to the floor slowly, keeping their feet connected on the floor.

4. Once on the floor, both partners scoot their hips as close to their feet as they can.

5. Feet and knees both stay hip-width apart and the heel lines up behind the second toe.

6. Both partners engage their abdominals by pulling their navel down towards the floor.

7. Keeping the strength in the belly, both partners lift their hips, then peel their backs off the floor one vertebrae at a time.

8. Both partners roll to the outside of their right shoulder, then to the outside of their left shoulder, clasping their hands underneath their back to add a chest opener.

   - If a partner needs additional support to hold the hips up, that partner can take the hands onto the backs of the hips instead of clasping them together.

9. The chin stays slightly away from the chest so the neck rests comfortably on the floor.

10. The eyes look straight to the ceiling; because the neck bears weight in this pose, each partner must keep the head centered and avoid turning the head.

11. Partner A lifts her left foot straight up to the sky as Partner B lifts his right foot straight up to the sky.

12. After both partners have a foot in the air, partners reach their lifted feet toward each other until the soles of the feet touch.

    • An option is for both partners to hold a solo Bridge pose next to each other, without the leg lift.

13. After holding for eight complete breath cycles, partners lower their feet, then lift the other leg to switch sides.

    • An advanced option is to have partners bring both feet together and lift both legs higher while their hands support the back, but they should attempt this only if they have been practicing solo Shoulder Stand for a long time and feel comfortable with Shoulder Stand; finding a comfortable balance point may require one or both partners to bend their knees.

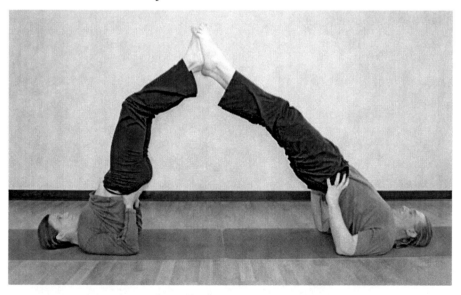

Drawbridge is a gentle inversion and a supported chest opener. This also strengthens the quadriceps muscles in the thighs. In this pose, you place the heart above the head, changing the normal gravitational resistance for your blood flow. This change of scenery does wonders for the mind as you look at the world from a completely different angle.

Symbolism: The symbolism in Drawbridge is in the inversion. We spend most of our day with our head above our heart, but in this pose we put our heart above our head. Though medically our emotions all stem from our brain, symbolically the heart represents our capacity for compassion. In Drawbridge we gesture that we place love above all else by placing our emotional center above our cognitive center.

This pose is a variation on Bridge *(Setu Bandha)*, and Shoulder Stand *(Salamba Sarvangasana)* in the advanced option.

Connected Rest

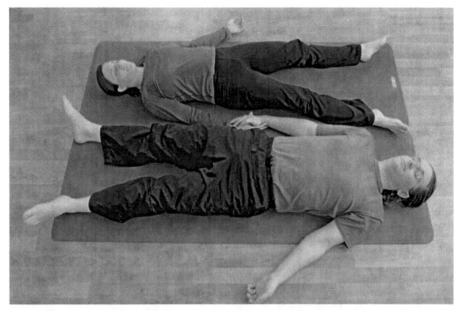

Connected Rest is the most important pose of the sequence because it's the pause button that enables the body and mind to absorb all of your previous work. Before coming into Connected Rest, both partners can grab their own knees and roll around on their backs a few times and twist side-to-side to work out any additional kinks before resting. Partners can also spend more time in Full Circle Breath before coming in to Connected Rest.

1. Both partners lie side-by-side with Partner A's feet by Partner B's head.

2. Both partners bring their inside hands to touch gently, letting the connected hands rest on the floor.

3. The outside hand rests on the floor a few inches away from the legs with the palms facing up.

    *   Another option is to have Partner A's outside palm up and Partner B's outside palm down, symbolizing the connection of upward moving *ha* (sun) energy and downward moving *tha* (moon) energy; the purpose of *hatha* yoga is to balance these two energies.

4. The feet stay several inches apart with the toes falling away to the outside.

5. Both partners lie still with eyes closed for several minutes enjoying the fruits of all their hard work.

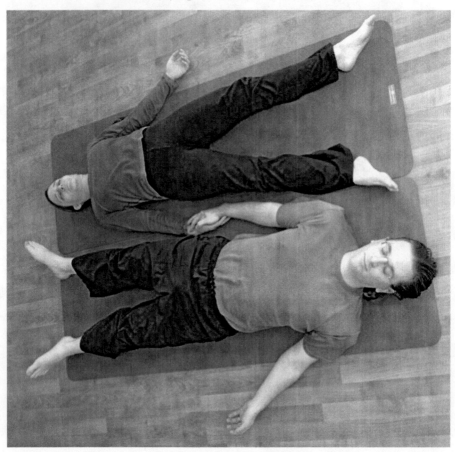

Connected Rest, a connected form of Corpse pose, is the most important pose in the whole sequence for two reasons. First, by lying still, your body has the time to record the muscle memory of all the strengthening and stretching, allowing you to reap the benefit of all the work in the poses. Second, the poses were initially created so that you can tire out the body enough to slow down the brain and rest for a while; in Connected Rest you enjoy that sense of rest.

Enjoy this well-earned downtime for your mind.

As thoughts drift into the mind, you can just let them drift out, without dwelling on any particular thought. If it helps, you can also count your breath, or focus on a visual image during this final rest. You can use the visualizations that we have provided in this book while resting in this pose.

Classically, people practice the final rest as a solo Corpse pose, but maintaining an effortless physical connection with your partner helps you share in the quiet together. It develops your ability to enjoy the company of people close to you without having to fill space with chatter or distractions. If you find yourself spending a great deal of your time with loved ones in front of the television, or with other distractions, then practicing this shared stillness and silence is essential.

By having one partner with the outside palm up, and the other partner with the outside palm down, you can symbolize receiving both the downward flowing receptive energy and the upward flowing aggressive energy in this pose. By having the hands connected, you share this energy between you, thereby balancing it.

Symbolism: The symbolism of Connected Rest is celebrating the level of comfort you have achieved when you and a partner can enjoy the quiet together.

This pose is a variation on Corpse *(Savasana).*

Suggested pose sequences

Here are some suggestions for pose sequences; you will, of course, come up with your own routines the more you practice.

Luxurious 90 minutes together routine

If you have this much time to spend on your partner practice, we suggest trying all the poses in this book in the order presented. After Connected Rest, you can use one of the visualizations to spend some time together in meditation.

Short wake-up routine

- Full Circle Breath
- Cat/Cow with a Starfish
- Upright Back Chair
- Open Hearted Warrior
- Double Down Dog
- Double Cobra
- Two Warriors
- Just Right Triangle
- Twister Triangle
- Full Circle Breath or Connected Rest

Wind-down routine

- Full Circle Breath
- Extended Table
- Double Tree
- Long Neck
- Open Cobbler's
- Diamond
- Child's Play

- Double Twist
- Connected Rest

Trust-building routine

- Full Circle Breath
- Arm Chair
- Double Angle
- Two Sided Plank
- Warrior 6
- Twister Triangle
- Pas de Deux
- Proud Sit
- Two Masted Boat
- Child's Play
- Connected Rest

Connection-building routine

- Full Circle Breath
- Cat/Cow with a Starfish
- Open Hearted Warrior
- Super Straddle
- Gibbous Moon
- Double Tree
- Double Straddle
- Forward Reach
- Lords and Ladies of the Fishes
- Drawbridge
- Connected Rest
- Visualization/Meditation

Friendship with oneself is all important because without it one cannot be friends with anybody else in the world.

—Eleanor Roosevelt

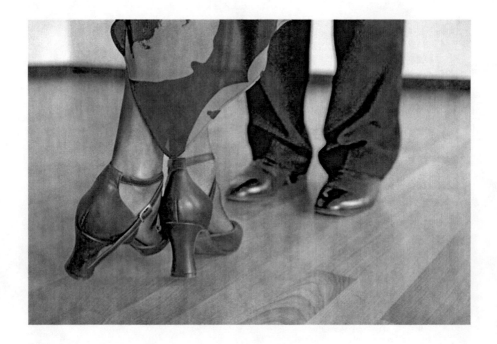

Visualizations, meditation, and deep breathing

Some consider meditation and visualization to be two separate things; we find them subtly distinct yet closely related, so we have grouped them together in this chapter. In the yogic tradition, visualization is akin to concentration *(dharana)*, and meditation *(dhyana)* is another limb of the eight-limb royal yoga system. They both are similar in that they require several minutes of sitting still using slow, deep, rhythmic breathing. Deep breathing is closely associated with another limb, called *pranayama*, but we find deep rhythmic breathing aids meditation so well that we have included it in this chapter.

In addition to practicing poses, adding some meditative practices to your routine will help you develop both the awareness, peacefulness, and stability that helps you form better relationships. Finding a few moments of quiet—not just physical quiet but mental quiet as well—helps recharge your psyche tremendously.

Note that meditative practices can sometimes cause you to face past issues, so it's possible that meditation can evoke strange emotional responses, dreams, and moods. Meditation holds a mirror up to our inner self and sometimes we see things we've tried very hard to ignore. Since modern society has so many distractions, we can spend days on end without any self-reflection, which makes a meditation practice so powerful. If you find yourself overwhelmed, seek counseling from either a professional or some trusted friends. Trust that you are not doing anything wrong if you have some mixed feelings after a meditation practice.

Deep breathing exercise

Steady rhythmic breathing is the key to a good meditation practice, just as it's the key to a good yoga pose practice. Before beginning your visualization or meditation practice, spend at least two minutes counting your breath without forcing it. As you move through your practice, keep coming back to counting your breath as a way to center yourself. We recommend doing a count of "inhale 1-2-3-4, exhale 4-3-2-1." The important thing is consistency of the tempo and the ease of the breath: it should never feel strained or rushed.

This is also a great de-escalation technique for when you find yourself in a heated argument—stop what you are doing and count your breath "inhale 1-2-3-4, exhale 4-3-2-1" for a few cycles. This will help you relax and will ensure that you are getting enough oxygen to your brain so that you can think clearly.

Deep rhythmic breathing is a simple and powerful tool you can use to reduce anxiety and maintain good communication with the people close to you. In less than a minute, deep rhythmic breathing can reduce stress levels in the body, making it an obvious and effective method for stress reduction.

Often people have very shallow breath, but when you inhale the entire torso should expand. The front, sides, and back of the chest should expand along with the belly. Allow your belly and chest to expand as you inhale and passively contract as you exhale. Try imagining a balloon inside the torso expanding in three dimensions as you inhale, then imagine it deflating evenly towards the center as you exhale. However, deep breathing should feel effortless, not strained, so keep the torso movements relaxed.

You can practice deep rhythmic breathing anywhere: on an airplane, while shopping, in traffic, just before an important meeting, before bedtime, etc. It's particularly useful for meditation and visualization practices.

Visualization exercises

Visualization is a great way to focus and de-clutter the mind. You can practice by yourself or with your partner. It's also a great practice to share to celebrate birthdays, anniversaries, etc. You can also use it to redirect your thoughts whenever you find yourself in a funk.

It can be done for as short as five minutes, or as long as hours. We strongly suggest blocking out at least twenty minutes in your day planner so you will not feel rushed. Visualization exercises also work very well after practicing the poses.

Arrange a comfortable seated position that enables you to maintain a long spine, such as sitting on a pillow with your back against the wall. If you practice simultaneously with a partner, you can sit facing each other, knee to knee, or back-to-back if you find that position less distracting.

Begin with your eyes closed, and count your breath "inhale 1-2-3-4, exhale 4-3-2-1" keeping an even steady rhythm. If practicing with a partner, you can begin with Full Circle Breath, but then eventually let your breath go on autopilot as you shift your focus to your visualization. When you feel your heart rate slow down, and your mind begin to focus, shift your concentration away from the breath and begin to work through the visualization.

We have two suggested visualizations here to get you started; you may want to ask your partner to read these to you the first time you practice. These visualizations are suggestions to give you ideas for creating your own.

Visualization 1: Long Lost Friend

Imagine your partner meeting up with one of her long lost friends. Imagine how she would describe you to her friend. Place your partner and her friend somewhere comfortable where they can talk, such as a park on a sunny day or a low-key restaurant. Visualize the whole scene of the conversation and put yourself in the vantage point of the long lost friend watching and listening to your partner.

Keep focusing on what your partner would say about you, not what you would say about yourself. Imagine the words coming right out of your partner's mouth. Hear with your mind her tone of voice, and the joy in her voice as she describes you. Listen to what words would she use to describe:

- Your personality

- Your achievements

- Your taste in food, music, movies, art, and literature

- Your hobbies

- Your sense of humor

- Your creativity

Now imagine your partner relaying her favorite memories to her friend such as a time when:

- You showed her kindness

- You showed her bravery

- You showed her forgiveness

- Your showed her loyalty

- You did something silly

- You did something wise

After you have gone through the visualization, write these words down and share them with your partner. See where in this exercise you let your own judgments come in and where you really allowed yourself to hear your partner's thoughts and words coming through.

Visualization 2: The Painting

Imagine your partner as a great painter. Imagine him painting a portrait of you. Visualize the technique of the brush strokes, see the colors used and sense the care and effort your partner is making to capture you. Focus on how he paints your physical attributes. Try not to add your own editorial comments into the painting but instead let his impressions come through.

Also imagine additional flourishes your partner would add to capture your essence or your personality—you can make the painting as wild and surrealistic as you want. Visualize some of the symbolism your partner uses to demonstrate how he views you in all of your complexity. See how your partner would capture your true nature visually.

After watching your partner create this portrait, begin to see this portrait as a mirror reflection of yourself. Embrace this image and imagine seeing yourself in this way. After your meditation session ends, write down what you saw so that you can come back to this visual when you need it. Notice points where you were able to truly see yourself for how your partner sees you and where you let your own perspective of yourself dominate.

An option for this visualization exercise is to visualize yourself as the painter and imagine how you would paint your partner. After your visualization session, share this information with your partner.

Create your own visualization practice

After practicing with your visualizations once or twice, you will undoubtedly create your own. Some people prefer audible cues during visualization, so you could even write a script and record it onto a CD. We suggest having someone else speak the script, because most people find the sound of their own voice distracting.

You can play some music during visualization if that helps, but avoid anything with lyrics, or anything with too many tempo or volume changes, because that can be disrupting.

Many thoughts and ideas will surface during a visualization practice, which is why we like the habit of keeping a journal. By writing down your thoughts after a long period of reflection, you can document your psychological evolution. We find journaling an excellent learning tool in general, but journaling after a visualization session is even more powerful because you can get deeper into your real thoughts and emotions.

Meditation practice

Meditation is slightly different from visualization and can take many forms. In visualization, the brain is focused, whereas in meditation, we let the brain relax. Often you will hear people say, "Just clear your mind," which is technically impossible because your brain is constantly receiving and sending signals from the rest of your body. Instead of clearing your mind, a better way to think about meditation is simply quieting your active mind, which means slowing down your thoughts. There are guided meditations or mantra-based meditations where you chant the same phrase over and over. A very basic form of meditation is just silently observing your breath. Practicing the yoga poses is, in fact, a form of meditation as well.

When you practice Connected Rest, you are practicing meditation. The important component of meditation is stillness. We don't allow much time for stillness in our society; sure we have lots of lethargy and couch-sitting, but that is different from stillness. Stillness means turning off the television. Just taking a few minutes of a time-out every day can help you better cope with the rest of your day. Many moms say that allowing themselves a few minutes of internal focus and stillness gives them the serenity to better deal with their children. Meditation recharges the battery bank of your mind.

Instead of worrying about technique, just try finding ten minutes a day of nothingness: no reading, no moving, no watching, no talking, no eating, no drinking, no listening, no nothing. Just spend ten minutes just being. Practicing this with a partner becomes a wonderful exercise in becoming so at peace with the presence of a partner you can surrender the vigilance of your active mind.

The ideas that have lighted my way have been kindness, beauty and truth.

—Albert Einstein

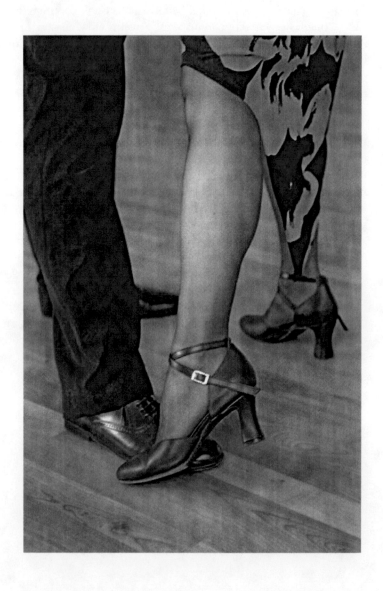

Applying yoga philosophy to relationships

So far we have discussed some of the limbs of royal yoga piece by piece, but here is an overview of all eight, so that you have a clearer picture of this practice. There are numerous texts out there that describe these limbs in detail, but we wanted to give you a basic primer on them, so you can draw some connection between the physical practice and the psychological practice of yoga. To study these in depth, pick up a translation of the *Yoga Sutras of Patanjali* with commentary.

In order, here are the eight limbs, or components, of royal yoga:

- *Yamas:* These are restraints, or the things we should not do in our day-to-day life.

- *Niyamas:* These are actions (literally, "not inactions"), or the things we should do in our day-to-day life.

- *Asana:* This tells us to find a comfortable seat, but yoga practitioners consider all kinds of odd positions to be comfortable seats, providing us with various yoga poses.

- *Pranayama:* Technically this means mastery of life force, but we generally take it to mean practicing various breathing exercises to regulate the flow of oxygen in the body.

- *Pratyahara:* This is withdrawal from the senses, which means bringing your focus inward, and not staying distracted by the sights, sounds, smells, tastes and sensations around you.

- *Dharana:* You can interpret this as concentration and focus, such as the concentration you use during the visualization practice. Many people practice this by repeating a mantra, or staring at an image.

- *Dhyana:* This means meditation, or the absence of distracting thoughts. The path to meditation usually leads first through withdrawal from the senses, then through focus.

- *Samadhi:* This is a state of unadulterated and unqualified bliss. Many people see this as a permanent state you reach after years of working on your yoga practice. Instead, we see it more as moments in pure bliss, and hopefully you can find more of these moments and learn to extend them.

The first two limbs—restraints and actions—deal with lifestyle and behavior, which makes them very accessible to us. There are five restraints and five actions that serve as guidelines.

Yogis believe that the teacher inside your own mind is the best teacher around, and that if you stop and listen to your own internal wisdom, you will learn a great deal. Some people refer to the restraints and actions as the Ten Commandments, but they are not so set in stone. Think of them more as ten golden rules, and remember that it's your job to give each of these some thought, and interpret them for yourself.

When contemplating the restraints and actions, keep the word moderation in your brain. Yoga texts often refer to "the middle path" whereby you walk evenly between two extremes. As you read these, imagine yourself finding that balance, or moderation.

You can find more discussion of these guidelines in various books, magazines, and Web forums. We hope to give you an introduction to how these apply to the realm of relationships. We hope that as you read our interpretations of the restraints and actions that you spend some time thinking about what they mean to you, and that these guidelines help you refine your own moral code. We strongly recommend discussing these with your partner as well, as you can often gain more insight by listening to how someone else interprets these guidelines.

Restraints

There are five restraints that serve as lifestyle guidelines. While these are considered the "don'ts" of yoga, we also like to look at the opposites, giving you some positive action to take.

Non-violence (Ahimsa)

In its most basic form, non-violence means refraining from physical violence, preventing others from being the victim of violence, and not allowing yourself to be the victim of violence. On a more subtle level, it means regarding and speaking to others with kindness, standing up for others, and treating yourself with respect.

We see two critical steps in applying the principle of non-violence to your existing relationships.

Treating yourself non-violently means treating yourself with compassion. When your partner hears you say, "I'm so fat/thin/old/stupid," you might as well be saying it to your partner. Words have impact and when you berate yourself you cause others around you to feel pain. We have all berated ourselves at one point or another, but working on self-talk is often step one. By creating a more positive internal dialogue, and treating yourself with kindness, you will be more open to treating others with kindness as well.

Step two becomes easier once you have worked hard at step one. Speaking to others with compassion takes work, especially when voices and tempers rise. Here's where deep breathing helps: it takes only twenty seconds of deep breathing to reduce stress hormones that pulse through our bodies, so the next time you find yourself ready to lash out verbally, try to take a few deep breaths. By pausing for just a few seconds, you can often regain your composure, and say what you really mean, rather than saying something mean.

Many resources offer training in de-escalation tactics and non-violent communication techniques, which can steer a conversation towards owning our reactions to our partner's behavior and asking for behavioral change in a positive manner. If you have struggled with conflict, we recommend taking a class in non-violent communication. These techniques will better equip you to behave with greater compassion in your relationships.

Truthfulness *(Satya)*

This principle tells us to refrain from lying to ourselves and to our partners. Truth is tough. One well-intentioned mistake that creates mistrust is when we tell the truth too late. Instead of trying to fix your partner's problems and shield him from unpleasant truth, involve him immediately in issues. When you cover up something, even when trying to protect your partner, you often do more damage because it communicates that you did not trust your partner to handle bad news with maturity.

This principle also means not lying to yourself. Many of us have had relationships—either romantic or platonic—that were far from nourishing. This principle informs us to recognize denial and to face problems with our relationships honestly. By using non-violent communication strategies, we can have more honesty in our relationships. By having more honesty in our relationships, we can have more non-violent communication.

Non-stealing *(Asteya)*

Non-stealing in a relationship means contributing equally. At the surface, we can evaluate this on a simple level of contributing equally to a relationship. For example, this means splitting the cleaning chores equally with your roommate and honoring the system of collaboration.

However, you can take it one step further with your roommate and offer to take over her duties when she is sick, without trying to barter with her to do double duty when she is better. You can simply look at it as right now, when she is sick, she is contributing all she can: she is not trying to steal your time by having you do extra work; she simply needs to heal.

Non-stealing also means avoiding jealousy. For example, you might resent the amount of time your spouse spends on an activity you do not enjoy, such as crossword puzzles, or fishing. Instead of harboring resentment, you can move beyond jealousy. First, realize that your spouse's enjoyment of an activity does not indicate any dissatisfaction with you. Second, appreciate the joy that activity brings to your spouse and be grateful for his or her happiness. Third, recognize that everyone needs some alone time, and take the opportunity to cultivate your own activities or enjoy your downtime and practice meditation. Finally, understand that often we harbor jealousy towards our spouse's activities because too often we have too little time. We often fill our lives with so much work that we have very little time to spend together. By carving out some real time together each week— time spent without the television to distract you, and doing an activity such as partner yoga—you can maintain your intimacy and not view the time your spouse spends on his or her hobby as wasted time. This can help you move beyond jealousy.

Continence *(Brahmacharya)*

Traditionally, people considered this restraint to mean celibacy. The original thought was that by abstaining from sex you hold onto your vitality and you can redirect that energy towards your yoga practice. Many yogis do in fact lead monastic lives. However, even the ancient texts refer to people called householders, which are people who have physical relationships with others, normally a spouse.

We view continence with the broader intention of maintaining your vigor. When we drink too much, eat too much, play too many video games, sleep too much, work too much, have too much sex, or even do too many yoga poses, we feel depleted. On a mental plain, when we obsess over things such as sex, politics, money, possessions, etc. we deplete our mental resources. So instead of viewing continence as abstention, you can view continence as constantly monitoring if you are doing something excessively to the point where it interferes with your vitality.

It may sound unoriginal, but moderation in all things is the best guideline for a healthy, vigorous life.

Non-greed *(Aparigraha)*

Non-greed is closely related to non-stealing. In fact, people steal out of greed and jealousy. We like to look at the other end of the spectrum from greed, and that is generosity. Generosity in your relationships means doing something for a loved one without expecting anything in return. Here are some examples of how to practice true generosity.

Offer to buy your friend dinner when he is out of work, without even thinking that someday he will return the favor. Even if he never is in a position to return the favor, opening your heart and showing compassion is its own reward.

When your partner looks like she is tense, stressed out, or just sore, offer her a neck massage or a foot massage, not in the hopes that she will give you one in exchange, but simply because you want to relieve her tension and stress. By acting out of true generosity, you will learn the wonderful satisfaction of purely helping others.

Actions

Some of the actions have a spiritual tone. However, practicing yoga is not adopting a new religion. When the yoga texts talk about god, it means whatever you personally believe in: be it Christianity, Wicca, or the exquisiteness of nature, or your love for your partner. The practice of these actions is a psychological discipline, one that better aligns your day-to-day life with your spiritual beliefs, whatever they may be.

Purity *(Saucha)*

Purity for relationships has both a physical and mental component. Keeping your household clean can reduce the stress and tension in any relationship. Dirty dishes sitting on the counter, dirty clothes lying around, and other messes all signal of work yet to be done which can cause stress. People normally have varying tolerances of clean, so it's important to establish right away what's important to each of you and try to respect those boundaries.

Purity also extends to how we take care of ourselves, including the quality of the food we ingest. In the West, our socialization tends to revolve around food and drink, and sometimes we view getting together with friends as an excuse to eat rich food, drink lots of alcohol, smoke various things, etc. Eating, drinking, and smoking with friends every so often is fine, but it is important to find other activities to do with them. Try arranging some different activities with your friends and loved ones such as: going for walks, taking adult education classes, visiting museums, learning a new dance, or going to a yoga class. By spending less of your socialization time eating, drinking and smoking, you can keep your diet more clean and healthy.

Purity of thought teaches us to avoid negative thoughts about our loved ones. Often these negative thoughts come from external sources: if we watch television shows where couples snipe at each other constantly, we can be trained to think that is normal behavior. Just stop sometimes and notice the effect of what you watch and read has on your thought process. One excellent way to clean your mind is to go on a media fast, where for one week you abstain from television and the Internet, and then observe any changes in your thoughts and behavior. We, of course, do not recommend permanently avoiding the news, as you need to know if your area is being evacuated because of wildfires or other such hazards, but you can also judiciously consume the news and avoid reading gossip and focus on more substantial things.

Contentment *(Santosha)*

Contentment teaches us to accept our friends as they are, rather than as we think they should be. No one can conform to an idealistic view of the perfect friend or the perfect mate. We are not saying to accept egregious or dangerous behavior, but we are saying to accept that everyone in your life is a work-in-progress. We are all working on our own challenges, and instead of dwelling on minor things you don't like, focus on the ways in which they enrich your life.

Of course, this doesn't mean that you stay quiet when you see people you care about in destructive situations. However, when you confront them you should accept that they may not change any time soon, so be grateful for any amount of good that they have brought to your life, especially if their reluctance to change means you part ways.

Contentment also teaches us to be happy with ourselves. Often people believe that once they find a mate they will be happy, but to find happiness in a relationship, you must first find happiness in yourself. The visualization exercises that we provide in this book can help you take inventory of your best qualities. You do not need a romantic partner to practice them, in fact, you can visualize your friends, your mother, or someone else describing or painting you. The more you practice positive self-reflection, the more you can find contentment. The more you can find contentment with yourself, the more you can extend it to everyone in your life.

Commitment *(Tapas)*

Commitment of marriage, or of friendship, takes determination and willpower. If you find yourself unable to commit your time to people in your life, you need to really examine your aversion: is it fear, laziness, or are you avoiding something that you know is truly not right for you to do? By practicing truthfulness, you will learn to commit to only those things that are truly beneficial and then adhere to those commitments.

Many people fret about not being able to commit to a relationship, but instead of fretting, start by examining your commitments to other people in your life. Do you follow through with helping friends when they move, calling your parents when you say you will, obliging on promises to visit, completing courses and projects, etc.? If the answer is no, stop and examine why you have a general commitment phobia; if the answer is yes, then it's probable you just have not found the proper match for that relationship. By working on your own honesty, sense of contentment and esteem, and by making commitments to yourself, you will soon find yourself open and ready to commit to the right person, if that is what you seek.

If you are in a committed relationship, recognize that commitment takes strength. This principle translates to fire, and it's the fire in our belly that powers our commitment. Practicing partner poses on a regular basis is an excellent example of commitment. By committing to practice yoga together, you are strengthening your commitment to your relationship.

Spiritual study *(Svadyaya)*

You can interpret this action as taking time to study or to practice your own religion, or whatever you consider special and important. Spending time together studying something you both consider sacred, such as attending church, or watching a sunset, keeps partnerships and friendships strong.

Since an overarching principle of yoga is that you are ultimately your own best teacher, spiritual study also teaches us to spend time in quiet reflection, or meditation. You don't need to contemplate the mysteries of the universe, though that is certainly interesting, but reflecting on what you have learned is very valuable. We suggest taking some time to meditate together; it can be very profound to share the same silent practice together.

One practice in yoga that you might find useful is to journal. Those who keep journals are always amazed when they read things they wrote even six months prior. Logging your thoughts is a great way to study your own mental or spiritual development. We have started a Christmas Eve tradition: Kimberlee writes in a special Christmas-Eve journal any fond memories she has of Todd over the past year, and things about him that she loves. When she is done, Todd writes about his reflections of Kimberlee and what he loves about her in the same journal. This is a wonderful tradition because we've been able to see our relationship evolve over the years, and reading this journal every Christmas is the most exceptional present by far.

Surrender to the divine *(Ishvar Pranidhana)*

You can interpret surrender to the divine means devoting your life to your religious beliefs. We also see it as putting the needs of those you love, such as your children, spouse, parents or friends above your own needs. By placing care of others above your own ego, you are, in fact, practicing compassion, or generosity.

True compassion—when you seek to help someone without any thought given to what you might receive in return—is perhaps the best example we have of surrendering yourself to the divine.

Overcoming obstacles

Yoga philosophers say there are five obstacles *(kleshas)* that we must overcome to attain liberation. These obstacles are also obstacles to having healthy, fulfilling, and yes, liberating relationships. We will briefly illustrate how you can examine your own behavior and recognize any of these behavior patterns. Becoming aware of a behavior pattern is the biggest step towards growth.

Ignorance *(Avidya)*

Know thyself. Through yoga, we work towards being free from the shackles of painful memories; this of course can take years. The first step towards healthy relationships is being cognizant when we repeat certain behaviors or when we transfer the blame of past injustices onto our current circle of loved ones. Many scars of childhood issues, along with friendship or romantic partnership breakups, can cloud our current judgment.

When you find yourself extraordinarily upset at a situation, stop and ask yourself, "Does this remind me of anything?" Scan your consciousness to remember the last time you felt that way. Quite often a very minor incident can evoke the pain of major one and we find ourselves overreacting. If you take the time to stop and recognize that something still haunts you, you can begin to address it. By becoming aware of your behavior and your reactions, you can discern the present from the past. This enables you to overcome your ignorance of what causes you to react in certain ways and allows you to deal with the present situation of your relationships.

By seeing your mate or your friends and the current issue for what they really are, rather than what memories they might evoke, you will find your communication far less defensive and hostile and far more positive and supportive.

Ego *(Asmita)*

Many things upset our ego, such as not being chosen as the maid of honor or best man at our friend's wedding, or recognizing that your spouse really does want to spend Saturday night with some friends. Our ego wants to think that we are the entire universe to all those in our orbit. At some point, all of us have gotten upset about unintended slights because of our ego. By identifying when your pride as been hurt, you can better separate the trivial slights from real injustices.

Practicing yoga and meditation can help us tame the egotistical beast. The more we learn that we have the power to be happy, regardless of circumstance, the more we develop a sense of self-security. This sense of self allows us to view the world, not through the lens of an ego that needs a constant stream of external validation to survive, but rather through the eyes of someone with a solid foundation of who they are, one that is timeless and one that cannot be injured by minor slights. Other people perceive us in their own way, but their perception is influenced by all of their past memories; by acknowledging this fact, we can recognize that what they see is not truly who we are. Our ego is concerned with what they see, but through practicing yoga, particularly meditation, we will see ourselves for who we really are.

Attachment to pleasure *(Raga)*

We love to feel good, but relationships require constant tending. Sometimes you need to have difficult talks with your loved ones to honestly face issues together. These talks are not fun, which is why some of us take what we believe to be the easier path of denial. Some people have an unrealistic expectation that if two people are meant to be together they will never disagree or argue. While you can discuss situations in a rational, loving and empathetic way, recognize that no two people have lived the exact same life, so you will inevitably interpret certain things differently.

So instead of denial, you can work on a strategy for how to disagree, and come up with some mutually-defined rules of engagement so that you can solve your problems as a team, rather than as opponents.

Attachment to pleasure can also manifest in avoidance of work. Everyone wants to spend their weekends relaxing and doing things they enjoy but, as many mothers have put it, "Trash does not take itself out." Instead of finding work a struggle, you can organize a schedule and responsibilities, so that you do not spring chores upon someone who has just started to read a book, practice yoga, etc. Allow some flexibility for when your housemates really do need a break. If you find yourself the one who avoids chores, see them as a way to truly practice your yoga. Stay present and mindful as you work and notice all the sensations involved in household work. This attention to detail, even on a task you do not find pleasurable, is an exercise in concentration, which is one of the limbs of yoga.

Aversion to pain *(Dvesa)*

Fear of rejection holds so many of us back. Fear of rejection is of course tied in with our ego. The more we view ourselves as having an essence that transcends both pleasure and pain, and that we share this same essence with everyone else, the more we can see rejection as a very superficial thing. They are not rejecting you—they are only rejecting their perception of you at this one moment in time. Who you are, and what they perceive you to be, may not be the same thing.

You will face rejection at many points in your life, but rejection simply means you tried something. The moment you stop trying is the moment your aversion to pain has conquered you. We believe that hockey player Wayne Gretsky said it best: when asked how many shots on goal he regretted, he said that he regretted 100 percent of the shots that he didn't take.

Even when people are in a relationship, fear of rejection plays a role. Sometimes people will keep their ideas, ambitions and fantasies to themselves out of fear they will be rejected by a partner. This often leads to resentment.

If you experience this, try one day to ask your mate about something fun he or she has always wanted to do, then share your idea. Perhaps you can reach some sort of agreement. For example, we made a deal that we would take tango dance lessons together in exchange for going on backpack trips (Todd was leery about dance lessons, and Kimberlee was leery about sleeping in the woods). Though we had initial moments of displeasure and some setbacks, Kimberlee ended up enjoying backpacking and Todd ended up enjoying tango. If the compromise tactic does not work, then you can either try your new activity alone or with a friend while reassuring your partner that you are not taking a step away from your relationship, but rather a step towards simply learning something new.

Fear of death *(Abhinivesah)*

How fear of death holds us back from healthy relationships is not so much a fear of our own death, but rather a fear of loss. Some people avoid getting close to someone, because they fear the time when they will lose that person. This is a very powerful feeling and quite a rational fear because we can see the pain of a lost spouse or child on the news regularly.

Fear of death is perhaps the most difficult of all obstacles. Yogic philosophy talks about our true essence as being eternal, and not bound to our physical body. You can interpret this to mean that at some level, you will always be connected to the people you love in spirit. This may provide comfort, but there are other yoga teachings that can help as well.

Yoga teaches us to embrace every moment, and realize that we cannot control the future, nor can we reconstruct the past. All we can do is live in the here and now. You can also view it by looking back to your childhood friends, whom at the time you thought were essential to your existence. As you aged, you slowly drifted apart from some of them, but you know that at the time, you were glad to know them. We can only trust that when the time comes to separate from our loved ones that we will feel true gratitude for the time they devoted to us. If anything, our fear of death can be a lesson to live in the present, and neither dwell upon the past nor fret about the future.

Namaste

You will hear the word *namaste* at the end of many yoga classes. Namaste has been translated in numerous ways; our favorite translation of this term is "I honor the place in your soul that has the same inherent goodness and light as I find in my own soul."

There is a powerful philosophy behind the term in that it deals with the concept of the true self, called *purusha* and the illusory self, called *prakriti*. You can view purusha as a very basic and pure essence that dwells within each of us, and prakriti as the labels and preconceived notions we project onto others. So when we say namaste, we are saying that we can see that pure essence (purusha) in someone else and that we recognize that pure essence as the same essence as within ourselves.

> "But without any identifications who are you? ...If you detach yourself completely from all the things you have identified yourself with, you realize yourself as the pure 'I.' In that pure 'I' there is no difference between you and me."
> —Sri Swamai Satchidandanda, *The Yoga Sutras of Patanjali*

By seeing your own pure essence and seeing that very same essence in your friends, you can begin to minimize expectations and preconceived notions, which clears the way for a more open dialogue and understanding. This is certainly a process, but through minding your behavior and practicing meditation, you can gain this insight. In your daily activities, try to examine if you are communicating with your loved ones through filters of labels. Are you reacting to them as, for example, a father—one whose definition has been shaped for you by your parents, your extended family, friends, television, books, movies, etc.—or are you reacting to them as someone who shares your very essence? What are your expectations from them? This is not a prescription for instant behavior change, but rather something to keep in mind throughout your life.

You can try this meditation practice that can help you see your partner as sharing the same pure essence as yourself. Stare at your partner for a while, then close your eyes and begin to see the edges of your partner's frame erode into just a glow of white light. Coming to a higher observation level, see yourself as the same glow of white light. Finally, see your two lights morph into a single glow of pure white light. After several minutes of this exercise, keep your eyes closed, bring your hands to your heart and bow as you say "namaste."

Each friend represents a world in us, a world possibly not born until they arrive, and it is only by this meeting that a new world is born.

—Anaïs Nin

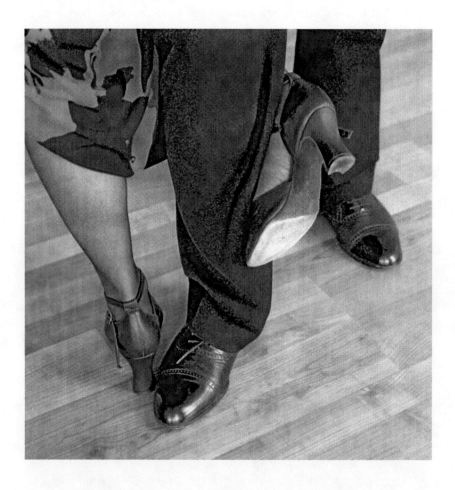

Next steps

We hope you have enjoyed our *Yoga with a Friend* book and hope this gives you a good baseline to begin a partner yoga practice. We encourage you to practice the poses in this book and to seek out a yoga class in your area and attend regularly. We have found that there are many partner yoga classes around, so if there is one in your area you should try it.

You can use this book as a sequence from start to finish, or you can simply pick and chose some poses. We actually believe practicing one or two partner poses with a friend or family member is a better way to introduce yoga to that person than taking him or her to a class. Going to a class is a time commitment—it involves scheduling, transportation, etc., whereas spending ten minutes doing some poses in the living room is nothing. The next time you are with your mom, dad, or whomever you have been encouraging to do yoga, ask them to try a few partner stretches with you.

Many people feel much more comfortable trying something new if they try it with someone they trust. By working with your friend in each pose, you provide confidence as that person tries something new and potentially intimidating.

Even though we demonstrate the poses with just one practice mate, you can certainly have some fun and creativity with the poses and find ways to incorporate several people in one pose. Be creative with your practice and enjoy the process of discovering new ways to move together.

Are we not like two volumes of one book?

—Marceline Desbordes-Valmore

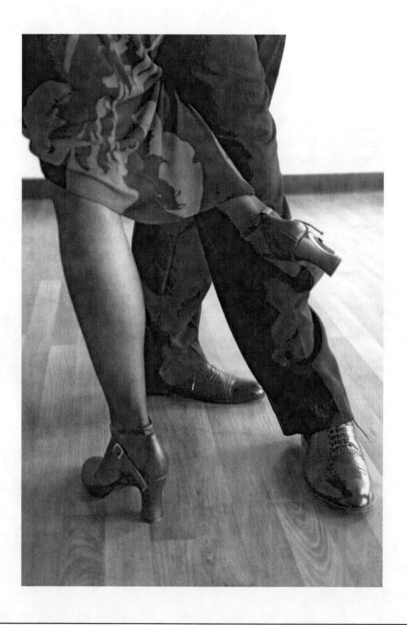

Resources

The following resources may help you develop your own practice. There are numerous resources on yoga out there, but here's a quick list to get your started.

Books

Anatomy of Hatha Yoga: A Manual for Students, Teachers, and Practitioners by H. David Coulter

Partner Yoga by Cain Carroll and Lori Kimata, N.D.

The Yoga Sutras of Patanjali translation and commentary by Sri Swami Satchidananda

DVDs

A.M. and P.M. Yoga for Beginners starring Rodney Yee, Patricia Walden, and Steve Adams

Partner Yoga starring Kate Mosley and Fiona Mays

Web sites

8th Element Yoga: www.8thElementYoga.com

Acro Yoga www.acroyoga.com

Punk Rock Yoga: www.PunkRockYoga.com

Yoga Basics: www.YogaBasics.com

Yoga Journal Pose Library: www.YogaJournal.com/poses/

Where there is love there is life.

—Mohandas K. Gandhi

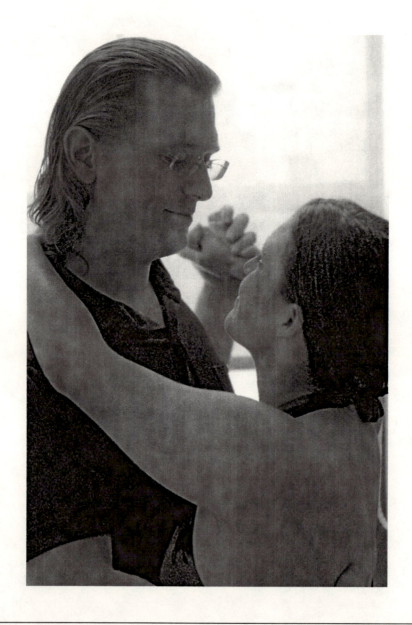

About the authors

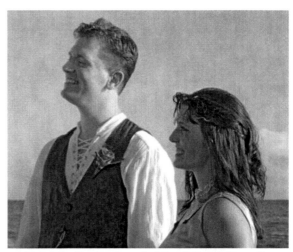

Kimberlee Jensen Stedl is a certified yoga instructor (200-hour Registered Yoga Teacher with the Yoga Alliance). She is certified in the YogaFit® style, and has experience in a variety of yoga disciplines such as Iyengar, Viniyoga and Kundalini, having practiced since 1997. Kimberlee founded Punk Rock Yoga®, an international yoga movement, in 2003. Kimberlee is a member of the American Council on Exercise (ACE) Continuing Education Faculty and has been an ACE Certified Group Fitness Instructor since 1992. She is also a certified group fitness instructor through the Aerobics and Fitness Association of America. Kimberlee established 8th Element Yoga (www.8thElementYoga.com) to support her diverse yoga interests. Kimberlee has a bachelor's degree in Journalism.

Todd Stedl is an Open Water Scuba Instructor certified through the Professional Association of Diving Instructors (PADI). He has been a dive professional since 2002, assisting as a divemaster for numerous instructors before becoming an instructor himself and establishing 8th Element Diving (www.8thElementDiving.com). Todd began his yoga journey in 2002, when he met Kimberlee and she used him as her practice student while attending teacher training. Todd holds a doctorate in chemistry from the University of Washington and has been a professional writer since 2000.

Together, Kimberlee and Todd have led workshops in the Seattle area that teach yoga with a friend. Besides yoga, they share numerous other passions, such as Argentine tango, which, like partner yoga, requires excellent non-verbal communication skills.

For questions, or to invite Todd and Kimberlee to present a workshop or retreat, contact us at DoYoga@8thElementYoga.com.

Printed in the United States
106984LV00007B/159/P

9 780615 183183